Hospital
Labor
Markets

Hospital Labor Markets

Analysis of Wages and Work-Force Composition

Frank A. Sloan
Bruce Steinwald
Vanderbilt University

LexingtonBooks
D.C. Heath and Company
Lexington, Massachusetts
Toronto

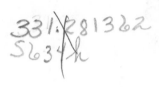

Library of Congress Cataloging in Publication Data

Sloan, Frank A
 Hospital labor markets.

 Bibliography: p.
 Includes index.
 1. Hospitals—Staff—Salaries, pensions, etc.—United States. 2. Hospitals—United States—Staff. I. Steinwald, Bruce, joint author. II. Title.
RA981.A2S548   331.2'81'362110973   79-5324
ISBN 0-669-03385-5

To our fathers,
Harry and Osmar

Contents

List of Tables

Acknowledgments

Like most empirical research projects, this book reflects the efforts of several individuals, and we would be remiss if we did not thank at least some of them. Our programmer was Ned Becker. The manuscript was typed by Dellinda Henry and Nanette Fancher, who added even tempers and tactful suggestions regarding grammar to their abundant secretarial skills. Several individuals, mostly Vanderbilt undergraduates, assisted in coding and other data-related tasks. We thank them collectively. The manuscript was edited, quite ably in our view, by Valeda Slade.

We are indebted to the Vanderbilt University Personnel Services Department for releasing to us the data used in the analysis of hospital wage scales in chapter 6.

Work on this project was initiated at the University of Florida, and some later data processing was also done there. John Wayne, who is currently at the University of Alabama, Birmingham, assisted in assembling the data files when he was a graduate student at the University of Florida. Richard Elnicki provided emergency aid in monitoring some large computer runs performed at the University of Florida's computer center for the empirical analysis in chapter 4. We are grateful to both of these individuals for their help.

This book represents a major part of the output from a grant to Vanderbilt University entitled "Determinants of Hospital Wage Inflation," grant number 5 R01-HS02590 from the National Center for Health Services Research (NCHSR), Department of Health, Education, and Welfare (DHEW). Linda Siegenthaler was our project officer. We thank her for her assistance throughout the project. A preliminary version of chapter 4 was presented at an NCHSR conference in early 1978, from which several valuable comments were obtained.

Finally, the conclusions expressed in this book do not necessarily reflect the views of NCHSR, Vanderbilt University, or any other agency or individual apart from the authors. Similarly, while we are grateful for all assistance and suggestions received, any errors in data, method, or interpretations are solely our responsibility.

1 Introduction

The Policy Context

By any standard, the growth in hospital costs has been dramatic. Between 1966, the year Medicare and Medicaid were introduced, and 1976, hospital expenditures rose from $14.2 billion to $55.7 billion, an increase of 292 percent. Even adjusted for the general rise in prices, expenditures more than doubled over this period. While part of this increase reflects both growth in utilization and provision of new services, the notion that large-scale expansion of hospital services is in itself desirable is now being questioned almost universally. With hospital expenditures accounting for 3.3 percent of the gross national product in 1976,[1] control over the rise in hospital costs must be seen as part of an overall strategy to restrain the U.S. inflation rate that has prevailed throughout the 1970s and to relieve pressures on budgets at all levels of government.

When confronted with such dramatic trends, there is a tendency to look for the villain. In a defensive stance, the hospital industry, like any number of other industries, places the blame on external causes. Causes frequently cited include inflation in prices of hospital inputs, greater unionization activity, rises in both the extent of minimum wage coverage and minimum wages themselves, tightening labor markets, the malpractice insurance crisis, and costs of complying with regulatory requirements.

Assessments by some presumably detached observers of developments in the hospital sector have been quite different. One relatively early view emphasized the predominance of nonprofit organizations in this sector. It was argued that such institutions are less cost conscious, and hence, less likely to be managed efficiently; furthermore, they more frequently engage in activities that, while perhaps socially desirable, are unprofitable. Taken in isolation, this line of reasoning provides a better explanation of the level rather than the rise in hospital costs.

The second and third explanations relate to factors determining the demand for the hospital's product. The growth in health insurance coverage and real per-capita income, especially during the latter part of the 1960s, is thought to have stimulated demand for hospital care. As of 1977, private and public third-party payments accounted for 94.1 percent of total payments to hospitals (Gibson and Fisher 1978). It has been maintained that greater patient ability to pay has improved hospitals' financial positions, thereby allowing them both to engage in uneconomic purchases of costly technical equipment and to pay their

1

employees more than they could earn elsewhere. This explanation complements the first by providing a reason for high rates of growth in real hospital expenditures.

The third explanation focuses on the role of physicians in determining demand for health care services in general, and hospital services in particular.[2] The physician is seen as the gatekeeper of the health care system. His advice and consent are needed before a patient can be admitted to the hospital, receive care from specialized units, or even purchase prescription drugs. Without taking a position on whether—or the extent to which—physicians shift demand for health care services, one can argue that increased physician availability has stimulated the demand for health care, including hospital services. Even if physicians are unable to shift demand for their product, greater doctor availability may cause the time price of health services to fall. The associated movement along the demand curve for physicians' services causes a shift in demand for the inputs physicians use in treating patients, including hospital care.

It is possible, and even likely, that there is some merit to all of the preceding explanations. One need not deny that events on the supply side have boosted factor costs while at the same time allowing a role for increased demand to affect input utilization and prices. Yet empirical differences in the relative magnitudes of supply- and demand-side influences as source of hospital cost growth do have important implications for public policy. For example, the case for hospital regulation—as a means of cost containment—is strengthened by empirical support for the demand view. On the other hand, to the extent that such supply side factors as minimum wages and aggressive unions are responsible, policymakers face a political dilemma. Any rollback of recent gains, such as the 1974 amendments to the National Labor Relations Act that extended the act to cover employees of nonprofit hospitals, would be seen by many as antilabor and against the "little man." But there may be a price to pay in terms of inflation.

One convenient way to describe the hospital cost inflation process is to consider the growth in four components: quantities and prices of labor and nonlabor inputs.[3] Using this descriptive approach, one might be able to rule out certain possible causes. For instance, if real wages were relatively constant over a given time period, it would be difficult to blame labor market-related factors. A shortcoming of this approach is that the comparative importance of the growth in individual components has varied over time, and the descriptive approach in itself does not ascribe reasons for these changes. Most recently, increases in the price of nonlabor inputs purchased by hospitals have been a cause for concern, reflecting in part the rise in energy and malpractice insurance rates.[4] But one may well question whether these particular trends will persist. Further, labor-related costs are the dominant ones in this industry. In short, all of these cost components merit attention by researchers; analytic investigations have the potential of shedding light on root causes.

Even though we stress cost containment, another general policy objective pertains to employment, particularly of women and ethnic minorities. The hospital industry is important in terms of the numbers of persons employed—by one account, 3.6 million as of 1977, or 4 percent of the civilian labor force, of which 76 percent are female and 18.9 percent are minorities.[5] Both the female and minority employment proportions are far higher for the hospital sector than for the U.S. economy as a whole.[6] From the vantage point of labor expenditures, what is a cost to third-party payors and ultimately to consumers is at the same time a payment to suppliers of labor and, in a considerable fraction of cases, to persons from economically disadvantaged segments of our population. Thus although high wage payments may be regrettable from the standpoint of the cost cutter, they benefit hospital employees. Irrespective of labor's contribution to hospital costs, the hospital sector contains many issues important for manpower policy, as well as for the distribution of employment opportunities and income.

Some recent studies of hospital costs in general, and hospital labor markets in particular, have stressed the rapid growth in both hospital employment and wages.[7] Our reading of recent trends, using essentially the same data sources, but in some cases more current data, is somewhat different. Detailed descriptive and multivariate analysis are presented later; however, at the outset, a review of some factual detail is useful to place this study in proper perspective.

Table 1-1 presents trends in employment and earnings for the U.S. economy as a whole and for selected sectors, including the hospital sector. The employment section of the table contains estimates of total employment, manufacturing and services employment, and three series on hospital employment. The first row of hospital estimates, like those of nonhospital employees, is based on *Employment and Earnings* (*E&E*) household data and covers employees in all hospital settings. The second hospital series, based on *E&E* establishment data, only pertains to nonsupervisory employees of private (nonprofit and proprietary) hospitals; the third series is from the American Hospital Association's (AHA) annual surveys of hospitals. It is not surprising that the second hospital series is the smallest. In principle, the first and third should coincide. That they do not probably reflects the different ways the two series were collected (from households and hospitals, respectively), methods used to impute missing values, and sampling errors.

Comparing the first hospital employment series with manufacturing and service sectors, it is evident that manufacturing employment was constant over 1970-1977. By contrast, service and hospital employment grew dramatically, with the service sector, which includes hospitals, rising at an even faster pace than the hospital industry alone. Using either of the other two hospital series, the comparative increase in service sector employment is even more pronounced. Certainly, the 1970s have witnessed a transformation in labor-force composition. In 1970, manufacturing and service sectors employed approximately equal numbers of persons; by 1977, the service sector had about 50 percent more

Table 1-1
Trends in Employment and Earnings

Industry	1968	1969	1970	1971	1972	1973	1974	1975	1976	1977	Growth Rate	
											1968-1977	*Other*
Employment[a]												
Total private	75,920	77,902	78,627	79,120	81,702	84,409	85,935	84,783	87,485	90,546	19.3	−0.5b
Manufacturing			20,737		19,866		20,879	19,275	20,044	20,637		51.1b
Services			20,266		21,749		23,041	23,759	24,829	30,629		28.3b
Hospitals[c]			2,841		3,026		3,269	3,394	3,568	3,645	61.8	44.8b
	1,543	1,638	1,725	1,791	1,821	1,879	1,987	2,293	2,388	2,497		22.5d
	2,309	2,426	2,537	2,589	2,671	2,769	2,919	3,023	3,108			
Hourly Earnings[e]												
Total private												
Undeflated	2.85	3.04	3.22	3.44	3.67	3.92	4.22	4.54	4.87	5.25	84.2	
Deflated	3.43	3.47	3.47	3.55	3.67	3.69	3.58	3.53	3.58	3.61	5.2	
Manufacturing												
Undeflated	3.01	3.19	3.36	3.57	3.81	4.08	4.41	4.81	5.19	5.63	87.0	
Deflated	3.62	3.64	3.62	3.68	3.81	3.84	3.74	3.74	3.81	3.87	6.9	
Services												
Undeflated	2.42	2.61	2.81	3.02	3.23	3.46	3.76	4.06	4.36	4.71	94.6	
Deflated	2.91	2.98	3.03	3.12	3.23	3.26	3.19	3.15	3.21	3.24	11.3	
Hospitals												
Undeflated	2.31	2.57	2.79	2.96	3.08	3.22	3.45	3.83	4.18	4.68	103.5	
Deflated	2.78	2.93	3.01	3.06	3.08	3.03	2.93	2.98	3.07	3.22	15.8	2.0g

Annual Earnings[f]

Hospitals							
Undeflated	5,921	6,529	7,051	7,368	7,787	8,635	9,336	57.7[g]
Deflated	6,380	6,745	7,051	6,938	6,605	6,709	6,860	7.5[g]

[a]Sources: *Employment and Earnings*, Establishment and Household Data; American Hospital Association (1977); U.S. Department of Commerce (1977).

[b]Growth rate 1970-1977.

[c]First row is for all employees, *E&E* Household Data; second row is for nonsupervisory hospital employees in private nonprofit and proprietary hospitals; third row is from annual hospital surveys conducted by the AHA and, like the first row, is for all hospital employees.

[d]Growth rate 1968-1976.

[e]Source: *E&E*, Establishment Data. All earnings figures exclude government employees and pertain to nonsupervisory employees. Deflated series are in 1972 dollars, using the Consumer Price Index as the deflator.

[f]Source: American Hospital Association (1976, 1977).

[g]Growth rate 1970-1976.

employees. In this sense, the growth in hospital employment is part of a more general phenomenon of growth in service employment.

Much of this book's focus is on wage determination in hospitals. Table 1-1 shows the broad earnings trends. In contrast to the 1960s, which were characterized by rapid growth in real income, from the employee's standpoint the decade ending in 1977 has been one of trying to preserve purchasing power. While real hourly earnings of nonsupervisory hospital employees in private hospitals increased 15.8 percent over the decade ending in 1977, this amounts to only 1.6 percent per year. The service sector as a whole was not much behind with an 11.3 percent real growth over the same period. Gains for the private sector as a whole and for manufacturing in particular, though positive, were negligible—about one-half a percent per year. Overall, the gains were sufficiently small that comparative growth rates in real hourly earnings are sensitive to the base and terminal years selected. For instance, considering 1970-1976, hospital employees fared worse than their counterparts in manufacturing and the service sector on the whole.

A series on annual earnings of hospital employees published by the AHA is also shown in table 1-1. Besides the difference in hourly versus annual earnings, this series differs from the *E&E*'s in encompassing (1) government as well as private hospital employees, and (2) supervisory as well as nonsupervisory employees, including physicians. The latter series demonstrates a 7.5 percent growth rate over 1970-1976 compared to 2 percent for *E&E* hospital employees over the same period. But the latter series implies that real hospital employee earnings reached their peak in 1972, a result confirmed by information from other sources, as is discussed in later chapters. By any measure, real earnings of hospital employees increased moderately during the past decade, far less than in the preceding one.[8] The four data bases analyzed in this study span the years 1960 to year-end 1977. Thus our charts and parameter estimates cover two widely contrasting periods.

Chapter Plan

Chapter 2 presents a conceptual framework for the study of labor markets, and markets for hospital labor in particular. Both the neoclassical model and some potential shortcomings of this model are discussed. We review distinctive characteristics of the hospital industry that have implications for the workings of hospital labor markets. Finally, the notion of philanthropic wage setting, a hypothesis first advanced by Martin Feldstein (1971), is introduced. Feldstein's hypothesis is evaluated empirically in chapter 4. Chapter 2 provides the general structure used in the next four chapters, which are organized by data base.

In chapter 3, hospital wage rates by occupational category, collected by the U.S. Bureau of Labor Statistics every three years, are analyzed to discern the impacts of changes in exogenous variables on both factor supply and demand sides of markets for hospital labor. As previously noted, the hospital industry has tended to emphasize developments on the factor supply side, while others, particularly economists, have stressed the role of demand. Chapter 3 sorts out supply and demand influences over the period 1960-1975. Among factors evaluated are the impacts of hospital unions, minimum wage legislation, and labor market tightness; the effects of various types of licensure and area amenities; and the role of increased third-party reimbursement and physician availability. Not surprisingly, some of both supply and demand classes of factors are found to be important hospital wage determinants.

Noting both the rapid rise in hospital wages during the 1960s and the fact that by the late 1960s and early 1970s hospital workers earned more in some occupations than their counterparts in other industries, Feldstein (1971) hypothesized that hospitals are philanthropic wage setters. Accordingly, hospitals have utilized some of their newly found revenue from third-party sources to pay their employees *rents,* that is, wage payments higher than required to attract them to hospital employment. Given that society has established other, presumably preferable, methods for transferring revenue to the disadvantaged, evidence that hospitals are indeed philanthropists in Feldstein's sense would have important ramifications for hospital reimbursement policies of third parties. Guided and perhaps armed with such evidence, government at both the federal and state level (the latter through insurance commissioners and rate review bodies) and, ultimately, private insurers themselves could develop methods to monitor wage payments.

The 1 percent public use samples of the 1960 and 1970 U.S. censuses are used in chapter 4 to assess empirically the notion of philanthropic wage setting. The analytic methods employed, though reasonably standard to economists, involve several steps that are described in detail in this chapter. On the whole, our empirical evidence is quite inconsistent with the view that hospitals have been philanthropists. Rather, a substantial part of the wage gains of the 1960s resulted from an upgrading of the hospital workforce. Of course, even descriptive evidence, such as that presented in table 1-1, would make it less likely that such a hypothesis would be proposed in the late 1970s. But our evidence implies that the notion is not particularly useful for describing the 1960s either.

Few would disagree that the most important government action affecting hospitals during the 1960s was the introduction of Medicare and Medicaid. By contrast, the 1970s have not witnessed the enactment of any new insurance programs. As noted previously, insurance coverage for hospital services is nearly complete in any case. Many of the more potentially important policy interventions during the 1970s have involved hospital regulation, including the Nixon Administration's Economic Stabilization Program, state certificate-of-need legislation, prospective reimbursement, and utilization review programs. Using a sample of 1,228 hospitals, based on annual surveys conducted by the American Hospital Association covering 6 years (1970-1975), we assess the role of various forms of hospital regulation on wage determination in chapter 5. The data base also permits us to reassess the impacts of several factors evaluated in previous chapters, including union effects on wages.

Since 1970, Vanderbilt University's Personnel Department has been conducting annual hospital wage surveys (with the exception of 1975). The sample is restricted to nonfederal, short-term general hospitals with at least four hundred beds. This wage information fills an important gap in existing data pertinent to hospital labor markets. Minimum and maximum wage information is available for seventy occupations, both health sector specific (for example, RNs, medical technologists) and more general (clerks, cleaners, and so forth). Union data are also available on a hospital basis from the Vanderbilt surveys and from the AHA. The last Vanderbilt survey reported in this study was conducted in late 1977, and thus provides our most recent information. Chapter 6, which presents our work based on this data source, is primarily descriptive, but it makes some assessments of the effects of the Nixon Administration's Economic Stabilization Program and contains some nonparametric tests of union impacts on wages. The latter analysis allows us to make some statements about the timing of union impacts. The descriptive evidence makes a useful contribution, in that recent occupation-specific wage data are available. This evidence is broadly consistent with the trends noted in our discussion of table 1-1. If anything, it implies that hospital employees have fared even less well than table 1-1 suggests, although low-wage hospital employees have made some gains relative to their more highly paid co-workers.

Chapter 7 summarizes our key findings, develops policy implications, and makes suggestions for future research.

Notes

1. American Hospital Association (1977).

2. For general discussions of physician-generated demand, see Newhouse (1978), Sloan and Feldman (1978), and Reinhardt (1978).

3. See, for example, Feldstein and Taylor (1977).

4. McMahon and Drake (1978).

5. All of these estimates are from *Employment and Earnings* (*E&E*) household data. See *E&E*, vol. 25, no. 1, January 1978. These points are emphasized in a recent report on health manpower policy by Fein and Bishop (1976). All *E&E* estimates in table 1-1 are also from this source.

6. As of 1977, the corresponding female and minority proportions for the economy as a whole were 40.5 and 10.8 percent, respectively. For manufacturing, they were 29.8 and 11.0 percent, respectively; for the service sector, they were 56.1 and 10.8 percent, respectively. See *E&E* source given in previous footnote.

7. See, for example, Feldstein (1971), Feldstein and Taylor (1977), and Taylor (1977).

8. See Taylor (1977).

2

Wage-Setting Models

Introduction

The study of variations in wages has a long history in economics. This is not to imply that a consensus currently exists as to the appropriate theory for analyzing labor markets and/or the interpretation of the substantial body of evidence that has been gathered. At the core of economics is the neoclassical model. Although simple, its predictive ability, in a labor context as well as others, is powerful. Yet many students of the field find important inconsistencies between the predictions of neoclassical economics and observed empirical behavior. In part, the controversy is the result of misreadings of the neoclassical position.

In this chapter, we first describe the standard neoclassical model of wage setting. Second, we consider ways in which hospital labor markets may conceivably depart from the standard model. Third, some more general criticisms of the standard model are discussed in terms of ways in which our analysis of hospital wage setting may be affected.

Wage Setting in a Neoclassical World

The neoclassical model provides a framework for describing causes of variations in quantities and prices. In the labor context, the focus is on employment and wages. Put simply, employment and wages are determined by factors operating on demand and supply sides of the labor market. But to say more, one must specify, among other things, (1) the length of the time period (that is, the *run*), (2) the structure of both product and factor markets (that is, the extent to which such markets deviate from the competitive norm), and (3) the assumptions about variations in worker tastes and nonpecuniary aspects of jobs that would account for wage differentials, even in equilibrium.

The notion of a run, describing the length of the time period considered by the analysis, is found in every microeconomics textbook. Even though the abstraction is relatively straightforward, difficulties arise in empirical application. In the neoclassical view, the employer's demand for labor varies directly with both the product price (or marginal revenue if the firm sells its goods or services in an imperfectly competitive market) and the worker's marginal product. In the short run, defined in part as a period too brief to permit large-scale movements of workers among employment settings and/or occupations, inelastic short-run supply largely determines the number of people in a given type of employment, while demand forces are the principal determinants of wage rates. With adequate time for job search, job changes, geographic mobility, and training, the labor supply curve generally becomes much more elastic. In fact, assuming homogeneous tastes, it becomes horizontal. With homogeneous tastes and a competitive labor market, but permitting differences in the attractiveness of various job attributes and other nonpecuniary factors, the compensation level is completely determined by the height of the supply curve, while the demand for labor curve determines the number of individuals employed.

Differences in the heights of the supply curves for various kinds of work and work settings are manifested in *compensating wage differentials*. These differentials reflect such factors as (1) the amount of training and experience required for the job; (2) physical and mental risks and the risk of losing the job during cyclical downturns; (3) attractiveness of the work environment, as well as the desirability of the area as a place to live; (4) area cost of living, if wages are measured in nominal terms; (5) fringe benefits; and (6) opportunities for subsequent work advancement because of job-related experience and/or connections obtained.

With heterogeneous worker tastes and/or nonreplicable skills, the long-run supply curve will have a positive slope, even assuming a competitive labor market.[1] The positively sloped labor supply curve will reflect variations in the asking wages of workers, arranged in order from those who like the work the most to those who like it the least. With a positively sloped long-run supply curve, wages depend on the strength of demand in both the short and the long run. The case of nonreplicable skills, at the extreme, leads to an inelastic supply curve, with demand for labor determining wages in both the long and the short run.

When monopsonistic elements are present, the employer faces an upward-sloping labor supply curve, even in the long run. Neoclassical economists have tended to dismiss monopsony as being inconsequential because they doubt that employers could maintain monopsonistic exploitation in the face of employee mobility. Yet its relevance to markets for specialized workers such as nurses or teachers (predominantly women), has certainly not been ruled out.[2] In any case, as already noted, the existence of monopsony power is not a necessary condition for a positively sloped long-run labor supply curve.

Neoclassical theory implies unambiguously that such forms of worker protection as minimum wages and trade unions tend to flatten portions of the upward-sloping labor supply curves and thereby, other things being equal, raise wages. Employment effects are less clear; under certain sets of conditions, minimum wages and unions may boost wages *and* employment of covered workers. Over the flat portion of the supply curve, wage rates are fully supply-side determined.

Licensure could conceivably create an absolute barrier to entry, whereby the supply curve becomes vertical at the amount of labor at which the restraint is reached. In practice, the stated objective of licensure legislation is to establish a minimum acceptable quality level. Additional entry requirements imposed by licensure authorities shift the supply curve in the covered occupation upward because the marginal entrant must secure higher compensation to recoup the higher entry costs. In this latter sense, licensure affects the position, but not necessarily the shape, of the labor supply curve. Other forms of regulation, especially those pertinent to hospitals, potentially affect wages by their impact on hospital demand for labor.

One's view of the general shape of labor supply curves is crucial to the empirical specification of wage equations. If one assumes horizontal labor supply curves, then only exogenous supply factors matter; changes in these cause vertical shifts in the supply function. Descriptors of job-related amenities (for example, working conditions) fall in this category. Exogenous forces on the demand side have no impact on wages when the supply function is horizontal. Studies explaining wage differentials in terms of differences in job-related risk (for example, Thaler and Rosen 1975) and amenities associated with a given job-residence location (for example, Getz and Huang 1978; Rosen mimeo), by excluding demand-side explanatory variables, are based on this assumption. The number of conditions needed to justify this type of specification makes it a special case. Allowing demand conditions to enter makes the analysis more general.

Failure to measure the role of demand-side factors in this study would foreclose an assessment of the role of third-party reimbursement and the bulk of potential effects of hospital regulation on wage determination in hospitals from the outset.[3] Even if the demand side plays no role in long-run equilibrium, this state of the world may be a long time in coming; and wage-setting trends in the short run may be dominated by demand-side phenomena. Therefore we include demand-side variables in our empirical analyses.

In all standard models of labor markets, the demand for labor curve is defined for the employing organization, generally a firm. Summing firm demand curves horizontally, one obtains demand for labor curves for the market area. For some types of work, the market area may be fairly circumscribed (for example, a city or part of a city); for others, especially skilled occupations, the market is national. Under perfect competition in the labor market, the wage is given to the employer. Hence, although the employer is free to decide how many individuals to hire as well as the skill mix of his work force, he has no power to set wages. It is appropriate in such cases to evaluate wage setting at a more aggregated level than the individual employer, such as a city. By contrast, the monopsonist determines both wages and employment, and, at least in principle it is appropriate to study wage setting at the level of the employer when one has ample reason to believe that monopsonistic elements are present.

Matters are by no means clear-cut in practice. One does not know shapes of supply curves in advance of empirical research. It seems reasonable to assert, however, that individual employers are wage takers for many types of laborers—the unskilled, for whom there are alternative employment opportunities in a locality; persons with general skills appropriate for a number of industries; and persons in highly skilled occupations for which interstate moves are the norm. This leaves a class of occupations, including nursing, for which geographic mobility for reasons of securing more advantageous jobs is fairly limited,[4] and for which job alternatives within the community are limited as well. But, local employer cartels aside, even persons in such occupations often have a number of job choices, especially in larger communities, such as major Standard Metropolitan Statistical Areas (SMSAs)—the observational unit in the wage analysis in chapter 3. In recent years, many investigators have favored using microdata as a means of avoiding aggregation bias.[5] For purposes of analysis of wage-setting patterns, however, a strong case can be made for using some kind of community as the observational unit.

Three out of four of the empirical chapters in this book use microdata on individual employees or individual hospitals as observational units for at least part of the analysis. How, in view of the preceding considerations, can this practice be justified?

In chapter 4, census data on individual employees are used to assess the amounts various types of employers, hospital and nonhospital, pay for workers with specific sets of characteristics. Without variations in these characteristics, detectable with individual employees as the observational unit, this part of our analysis could not have been undertaken. Later in the chapter, characteristic-specific wages are themselves the dependent variables with the state as the observational unit. This chapter thus does not depart from the notion that wage setting occurs at a community rather than hospital level.

To evaluate effects of specific reimbursement-regulation arrangements in chapter 5, American Hospital Association data on mean salary per full-time equivalent employee constitute the dependent variable, with the individual hospital as the observational unit. As defined, the dependent variable may be expected to vary principally because of differences in (1) area-specific wage rates, and (2) skill mix, which may vary substantially from hospital to hospital, even within a given community. Furthermore, we develop hospital-specific measures of union activity. As documented in later chapters, hospital unions rarely cover the whole community. It is therefore entirely possible that union activity may generate disequilibrium wage differentials within communities, although the market in the absence of unions is basically competitive (that is, wages in unionized hospitals may be above the equilibrium wage with more workers seeking employment in such hospitals than are able to secure jobs there). This in turn may depress wages in nonunionized hospitals, especially in hospital- and/or health-specific occupations.

The nonparametric analysis in chapter 6, based on Vanderbilt University's hospital wage surveys, also uses the hospital as the observational unit. An objective of this analysis is to assess union effects on wages, and the preceding reasoning applies here as well.

If it seems that we are not sympathetic to the monopsony hypothesis, we are conveying the correct impression. As argued in the next chapter, data appropriate for evaluating the hypothesis in a hospital context are currently unavailable. We question the validity of much of past empirical research on this topic for this reason. Also, if hospitals do indeed possess and exercise monopsony power, the concept applies to a few occupations at most.

Is the Neoclassical Model Appropriate for Analysis of Hospital Wage Setting?

To this point, we have described the labor demand curve in quite general terms. Yet the neoclassical model was developed under the assumption that firms maximize profits; it is nearly silent on such matters as product quality, output mix, and nearly vertical product demand curves due to the prevalence (and dominance) of third-party reimbursement. If hospital labor markets differ from most others, it is on the demand rather than on the supply (of labor) side. This section's discussion is cast in general terms. Elsewhere, we have shown in detail that the returns from developing formal (mathematical) models of hospital behavior are slim indeed.[6] The hospital, like any firm, must decide on the quantities of various types of outputs it desires to produce and the quantities of various types of inputs most appropriate to produce them.[7] For analytical purposes, it is convenient to assume that the hospital's output and input decisions are guided both by its objectives and the constraints it faces.

Profit maximization is most frequently assumed to be the objective of the firm in economic analysis. The single goal of profit maximization is inappropriate for most hospitals—the private nonprofit and government hospitals. But because hospitals may retain profits either to offset future losses or to make capital purchases, the pursuit of profits may be seen as one of several objectives rather than the single objective of the hospital.[8] Additional plausible objectives for the nonprofit hospital relate to the quantity of hospital services delivered, the quality of services (or their complexity or intensity), employment of particular kinds of workers and nonlabor inputs, emoluments to management, use of certain types of capital or labor inputs to enhance prestige, and payment of economic rents to workers, among others.[9] Alternative assumptions about hospital objectives do not greatly change the equations used in empirical analysis, but they do affect the power of the theoretical analysis to generate hypotheses for empirical testing. In other words, as goals are added, the complexity of the analysis rises exponentially. It is difficult to generate unambiguous predictions with as few as two or three objectives.[10] Plausible constraints on hospital decision making involve the technology of production (as reflected by a production function), a downward-sloping demand schedule for the hospital's services, exogenous factor prices, and, *possibly,* for a few labor inputs, upward-sloping labor supply curves.

Most models of hospital behavior incorporate one or more of the preceding objectives.[11] An exception is the Pauly-Redisch (1973) model of the hospital as a physicians' cooperative, basically a profit-maximizing model in which medical staff (attending physicians) run hospitals at least cost to maximize income to themselves. Pauly and Redisch have clearly made a conceptual contribution toward the understanding of a class of small- to medium-sized hospitals that may indeed be organized in physicians' financial interests. But it is difficult to see how their framework would apply to large teaching and/or government hospitals that, after all, are major employers. One should not rule out the applicability of hospital models that include various nonfinancial objectives. As a rule, the cost of realism is that many of the neat predictions of neoclassical theory, its most positive feature, are lost. Instead, directions as well as magnitudes of effects of exogenous demand and supply forces on dependent variables must be settled empirically. Knowledge of health sector institutions is an aid toward specifying which demand and supply influences to include.

Because this study focuses on hospital labor markets, possible hospital objectives relating to types of labor employed and levels of employee compensation merit special consideration. Hospital administrators may derive personal satisfaction from employing persons with certain backgrounds, for example, baccalaureate (BA) as opposed to associate degree (AD) RNs. The strict neoclassicist would find no inconsistency with this if the higher wage paid the BA were offset by savings in on-the-job training costs, greater flexibility, and/or higher productivity.[12] However, his theory would be disturbed by the administrator who hired BAs for the sake of his own and/or the hospital's prestige. Given such a reason, under competition the firm would be driven out of business; under monopoly conditions, the firm would be a buy-out candidate, since a profit-oriented purchaser could buy the firm, as currently operated, and make money by operating it more efficiently.[13] Whether administrators make employment decisions on the basis of prestige is a difficult, if not impossible, question to settle empirically. That a hospital employs a higher proportion of baccalaureate RNs may be a reflection of hospital case mix rather than administrator preferences. The productivity or greater flexibility of the baccalaureate RN may interact with case-mix complexity in subtle ways.

The notion that hospital wage setting is governed in part by philanthropic motives of hospital administrators has been advanced by Martin Feldstein (1971). It is conceivable that instead of, or in addition to, spending its surplus income on medical staff (as the Pauly-Redisch model implies), on emoluments to management, and/or on quality above that demanded by the market, hospitals transfer the surplus in part or in full to their employees.

Whether the hospital's motive is purely a philanthropic one or stems from a desire (1) to reduce employee turnover, (2) to improve morale, and/or (3) to improve employee productivity through increased job satisfaction, would be all but impossible to determine empirically. Administrators could hardly be expected to admit they are wage philanthropists, since such payments would not be considered "reasonable" by third-party payors. Feldstein developed the hypothesis to explain the rapid rise in real wages of hospital employees during the 1960s, coincident with a massive infusion of third-party payments due to the enactment of Medicare and Medicaid, as well as the fact that by the late 1960s and early 1970s, hospital employees in *some* major cities were paid more than their counterparts in other industries. But this hypothesis is inconsistent with two more recent facts about hospital labor markets: (1) the rapid growth of hospital unions, and (2) the decline in the rate of growth in real hospital wages and, in some cases (depending on the time period and occupation), the fall in real hospital wages during the 1970s. We conduct a detailed empirical assessment of the philanthropic wage-setting hypothesis in chapter 4.

Although interesting from the vantage point of basic research on hospital behavior, the philanthropic motive is not of central importance from the standpoint of policy, except, of course, if one objects to the use of cost-based reimbursement for achieving redistributional objectives. It is also of interest to know whether hospitals have used third-party reimbursement to pay more for a given set of worker attributes than even the high-wage industries, which have been identified in several studies. Another basic consideration is whether health insurance has changed the role of the hospital from "an employer of last resort"—that is, an employer that hires persons whose work histories include frequent job changes or periods of unemployment— to an employer that hires persons with characteristics similar to those employed by firms in traditionally high-paying industries. Although upgrading hospital work-force quality may be desirable from the standpoint of the hospital and persons specifically concerned about health care delivery, this development may not be seen as desirable by those concerned about employment opportunities of the disadvantaged or minority group workers who may now face new barriers to hospital employment.

Criticisms of the Neoclassical Model

In a neoclassical context, wage and employment levels reflect exogenous forces on the labor demand and exogenous factor supply sides. That we are dealing with a complex institution such as the hospital does not appear to destroy the usefulness of the basic neoclassical model. On the other hand, the neoclassical model itself has been the subject of a great deal of critical writing in recent years.[14] A few aspects of these critiques are enlightening in this context.

The challenge to neoclassical labor theory practically dates back to the publication of the comprehensive statement on neoclassical labor markets by Paul Douglas (1934). Certainly by the 1950s critical evaluations were widespread (Kerr 1950, 1954; Dunlop 1957). At the risk of oversimplification, there have been two types of critique. One stresses the simplicity of the neoclassical model's underlying assumptions and implied decision-making processes; the other claims that empirical evidence on labor markets is at variance with the neoclassical model's predictions. The second, if true, is far more devastating than the first.[15] That people individually do not act as the neoclassical model states they should can be discounted if the model proves to be a good predictor of market behavior.

Part of the second type of critique most closely related to our study (especially the census analysis in chapter 4) pertains to the persistence of interindustry wage differentials. According to neoclassical theory, interindustry wage rate differences should, in the long run, reflect only such factors as occupational mix, worker quality, working conditions, cyclical sensitivity of employment in the industry, cost of living in geographic areas in which the industry is predominately located, and the like. Variations in other factors, such as the firm's or industry's capital-labor ratio and product demand differences, should account for little or no interindustry wage rate differences, because movements from low- to high-wage industries may be expected to raise wages in the former, and lower them in the latter until equality or equilibrium differentials (solely because of working conditions, skill mix, etc.) are achieved.

However, specialists in labor economics and related fields have observed that interindustry differentials persist over long periods of time. Transactions costs associated with moving do not provide a full explanation of the failures of interindustry wage rates, especially those pertaining to a well-defined geographic area, to equalize over the very long run. As indicated more fully later, high wage rates are often found in highly concentrated, profitable, and unionized industries. Some studies show that a differential persists even after adjustments have been made for worker quality or skill mix.

Several writers have argued that industries in which monopolistic power has resulted in supernormal profits use these funds (sometimes under the duress of labor unions) to pay workers unusually high wages; that is, wages above the workers' opportunity costs. There are, however, several methodological problems with this argument. For example, persistently high profits may be associated with persistent expansion, and rapidly expanding industries may have to continuously offer relatively high wage rates in the short run to expand their work force rapidly.

But in spite of deficiencies such as this, the work of these researchers should not be dismissed out of hand. According to those who stress persistent interindustry wage differentials, a highly profitable firm derives several benefits from paying higher than "normal" wages: a greater selectivity in choosing employees; increased worker good will; less time spent in recruitment; reduction in turnover which is particularly costly where there is substantial on-the-job training; serving the philanthropic motives of the employer; and allowing the firm to keep wages reasonably constant over the business cycle.[16] To the extent that some items on the list are consistent with profit maximization, they may be consistent with the standard, neoclassical view. The selectivity and turnover reduction motives may fall into this category.[17]

Yet, if this is so, one is left with the question why firms in more highly concentrated and perhaps more profitable industries are more efficient users of labor inputs. One answer may be that causality really runs from efficient personnel policies to profits rather than the reverse, but this response may oversimplify a complex relationship. Philanthropic motives would seem to be inconsistent with profit maximization (unless one wants to argue that a better public image increases demand for a firm's product).[18] The desire to keep wages constant reflects the views of Galbraith (1967). Accordingly, large firms in concentrated industries typically plan price, output, and costs, far in advance. High and stable wage rates enable these firms to forecast production costs more accurately. Again, to the extent that such policies help minimize adjustment costs, they too are consistent with the standard theory.

A firm's ability to pay higher wages has been measured by the following types of variables:[19] industry concentration ratios; measures of past or present profits; wage bill as a percentage of value added; ratio of value added to the number of production worker manhours; ratio of male employment to total employment; and industry dummy variables to account for specific "industry effects." The concentration ratio and industry dummies are the most appealing (of a not very appealing list, in our view) on conceptual grounds. Profits, unfortunately, as we have said, may be jointly determined with wages. The male ratio is used as an ability-to-pay variable by Brown (1962) because "firms and industries which do not feel they can afford to hire prime male labor often resort to cheaper female labor and, therefore, employ lower proportions of men" (p. 48). When several ability-to-pay variables have been entered into an earnings equation, at least some always have had a statistically significant effect on wages.[20] Neoclassical economists would attribute industry effects to such factors as working conditions, job-related risks, prestige, and the like. Although the body of research by nonneoclassical labor economists is by no means flawless, it raises important questions that remain less than fully answered. Our empirical evaluation of philanthropic wage setting in chapter 4, which compares hospital wages with those in other sectors, assesses these issues once again.[21]

Critics of the neoclassical model consistently contend that the model is supply-oriented while most of the explanation of wage patterns lies on the demand side.[22] Defenders of the orthodox faith maintain that both supply and demand factors are essential to wage determination;[23] and we agree that the critics have misinterpreted the neoclassical view. Yet some studies in the neoclassical tradition, especially the "hedonic" wage studies that infer implicit price weights workers place on various nonmarketable attributes of the job itself and its location, by focusing almost entirely on the supply factors, give the critics' arguments some credence. It is difficult to believe that an emphasis on such independent variables as climate, crime rates, and job-related hazards can adequately account for movements of hospital wages or those in other industries, either spatially or intertemporally.

There is also controversy about the interpretation of specific employee characteristic variables in estimated earnings or wage functions. Do findings that blacks and women earn less, other things being equal, than their white and male counterparts reflect discrimination in factor and/or product markets, or another variable, not specifically included in the analysis, in some way related to worker productivity? According to the second view, the list of explanatory variables may be lengthy, but not lengthy enough. Persistent differentials in earnings and wages among various demographic groups, unrelated to productivity, are inconsistent with the competitive variant of the neoclassical model, as employers who persist in discriminating should be forced out by more efficient competitors. Under monopoly in the product market, persistent discrimination is possible under certain very restrictive conditions.[24] In this instance, the critics have a fairly good case; but with available data, sorting out the degree to which earnings differentials reflect "pure" discrimination is nearly an impossible task. In our study, this particular issue arises in chapter 4.

General Implications

This chapter, like the previous one, sets the stage for further analysis. The conceptual framework underlying the next four chapters is the neoclassical model of the labor market. Given the complex nature of the hospital, we do not present a model in formal terms, and the task of empirical specification awaits later chapters. The cost of dealing with institutions that on the average are more complex organizations than the prototypical firm of neoclassical economics is the loss of theory's predictive power. Although virtually any estimated coefficient can be rationalized in principle, we will, however, have more confidence in the analysis if the results are amenable to common sense interpretations. In any event, the ultimate objective of our empirical analysis is not to evaluate alternative theories of hospital wage setting, but rather to ascertain which policies and more general exogenous factors are chiefly responsible for observed trends in hospital wages.

Many issues have been debated by researchers specializing in labor markets, and no simple theory has emerged the clear victor. Although we find the neoclassical position to be somewhat stronger on balance than that of its critics, the latter have raised some important questions, based on observed empirical relationships, that have not been resolved to date. We cannot hope to resolve major controversies in the labor economics field in this study. Our goals are much more limited, and, given the aforementioned uncertainties, many of our results must be interpreted with both caution and a sense of modesty.

Notes

1. This point is developed in much greater detail by Rees (1973).

2. See Altman (1971), Cain (1976), and Yett (1970). We discuss the monopsony issue in greater detail in chapter 4.

3. We say more about the role of selected supply-side wage determinants later on.

4. For information on nurse mobility patterns, see Sloan (1975, 1978).

5. Discussions of aggregation bias are found in econometrics texts. See, for example, Maddala (1977).

6. See Sloan and Steinwald (forthcoming, 1980).

7. The hospital may also select a particular quality (of service) level that is reflected in derived demands for inputs.

8. Davis (1972).

9. This type of model assumes that the hospital can define its goals. Interesting goal conflict models (administrator versus trustees versus medical staff, and so on) may be realistic, but at the cost of additional analytic complexity. A model of this type is presented by Harris (1977). Economic rents are payment levels above the minimum required to attract an input to a particular use. For example, if a worker is willing to work 40 hours per week at $4.00 an hour, any weekly wage above $160 represents a rent.

10. This point has frequently been misunderstood by investigators in the field of health services research, including health economists. For additional discussion and evidence, see Sloan and Steinwald (forthcoming, 1980). Also, see Feldstein (1974).

11. See, for example, Evans (1970), Newhouse (1970), Lee (1971), and Ginsburg (1976).

12. Whether baccalaureate RNs are in fact more cost-effective is currently the subject of much debate in the nursing field.

13. See Alchian and Kessel (1962).

14. Reviews of the controversy in a labor context include Leibenstein (1974), Blaug (1976), Cain (1976), and Morley (1979).

15. In fact, many of the alleged structural inconsistencies, such as the presence of internal labor markets and the importance of custom in wage setting, are easily reconciled with the neoclassical model. See Wachter (1974).

16. See Brown (1962) and (for the last reason) Hammermesh (1972).

17. See Reder (1955) for reasons why a firm may set high wages to choose from a pool of qualified job applicants.

18. The philanthropic motive has also been ascribed to government em-

ployers. Fogel and Levin (1974) present some evidence that state and local government employers pay relatively high wages to low- and middle-level employees but not to top-level executives.

19. This list reflects Brown (1962), Eckstein and Wilson (1962), Kumar (1972), Stafford (1968), Wachtel and Betsey (1972), and Weiss (1966).

20. See the studies listed in note 19.

21. A somewhat more sophisticated institutionalist argument can be made using the concepts of key wage and wage contours. (The concepts are discussed in Dunlop 1957). In industries with a large percentage of females, the key wage is more likely to correspond to a "female" job. Female wages are likely to be lower for reasons of work experience, expected longevity on the job, and/or discrimination. The key wage by definition sets the wage pattern for employees in other occupations or skill categories. If the key wage is low, wages of other employees within the firm or industry are likely to be relatively low.

22. See, for example, Wachtel and Betsey (1972) and Bluestone (1970).

23. For example, Rees (1973).

24. Namely: (1) if monopolists are willing to lose profits in order to discriminate; (2) if barriers to entry preclude purchasing the discriminating firm by a nondiscriminating, and therefore more efficient, firm; (3) under regulation, when any additional profits from a nondiscriminating policy would be taxed. See Alchian and Kessel (1962). Evidence on regulatory effects on wages is just beginning to accumulate. See Hendricks (1977).

3

Hospital Wage Inflation—Cost Push, Demand Pull, or Both?

Introduction

There are two major competing schools of thought as to the reasons for the rise in hospital wages during the past two decades. The more traditional view, held by many in the hospital industry, is the cost-push theory. According to this theory, wage increases in the hospital sector reflect (1) a general tightening in labor markets in the U.S. economy as a whole; (2) the enactment of minimum wage legislation covering hospital employees at both state and federal levels, as well as subsequent increases in statutory minimum wages; and (3) the extension of collective bargaining enabling legislation to larger numbers of hospital employees and the ensuing rise in union coverage in this sector. Certainly few would maintain that labor markets have been tight during the 1970s (in marked contrast to much of the 1960s), but the minimum wage and union arguments are more plausible in the 1970s than in previous years.

Other potential wage determinants on the cost or supply side, less frequently mentioned by representatives of the hospital industry, relate to new health manpower training programs, changes in licensure requirements, and monopsony power. Health manpower programs have expanded dramatically in recent years—if anything, they should have offset other inflationary influences. However, these programs pertain to the professional segment of the hospital labor market and consequently have no direct bearing on wages of nonprofessional employees. Licensure of some types of health professionals has also become more widespread. In nursing, a field in which licensing has been universal for years, many states have changed from permissive (voluntary) to mandatory (compulsory) licensure. Under permissive licensure, unlicensed persons are not prohibited from working in the field, but they may not use the protected title; mandatory licensure prohibits unlicensed persons from working in the field.[1] Licensure in general may or may not improve the average quality of employees in the covered occupation. However, one can be sure that supply restrictions resulting from licensure in general, and mandatory licensure in particular, boost the wages of those in covered groups. By how much is an empirical question. Finally, to the extent that hospitals possess monopsony power, wages are lower than they otherwise would be. As argued later, determining whether hospitals in fact possess monopsony power in markets for certain categories of employees involves a number of complex issues. Because of

21

measurement problems inherent in gauging *levels* of monopsony influence, we are unable to state whether monopsony is more or less prevelant in the hospital sector now than in previous years.

A competing view of hospital wage determinants, held by several economists, emphasizes the demand side—especially the effects of increased third-party reimbursement and personal income.[2] Presumably, improved patient ability to pay raises demand for both quantity and quality (however defined) of hospital services, which in turn increases hospital demand for inputs. In the short run, at least, input prices should rise as a result. As noted in chapter 2, Martin Feldstein (1971) has extended this notion somewhat further, arguing that hospitals have used their improved revenue positions to pay rents to their employees. We deal with this conjecture in greater detail in the next chapter; therefore, we will not consider Feldstein's argument here. The demand variables used in the empirical analysis in this chapter do not permit one to distinguish between wage increases stimulated by the traditional demand mechanisms, and possible philanthropic behavior of hospitals induced by insurance and/or other demand-shift factors.

Conceptually speaking, both the cost-push and demand-pull theories of hospital wage inflation are consistent with a neoclassical theory of labor markets. At issue is which of the two curves has shifted the most. Many of the supply-side influences are beyond the health policymaker's control. On the other hand, the extent of health insurance coverage and third-party reimbursement policies are definitely subject to control.

The core data base for the empirical analysis in this chapter are the *Industry Wage Surveys of Hospitals* conducted every three years by the U.S. Bureau of Labor Statistics (BLS). Our analysis covers the period 1960-1975. Although previous research on hospital wages has been conducted with these BLS data,[3] our analysis encompasses a broader range of occupations—professional and nonprofessional, clerical and blue-collar—covers more years, and develops several new explanatory variables.

Basic theoretical considerations have already been discussed in chapter 2; hence, we move directly to a description of the BLS wage surveys and empirical specification in the next two sections. Empirical results are discussed in the fourth section. The final section summarizes our findings and considers policy implications. Applicable previous research is integrated into both specification and results sections of this chapter.

Bureau of Labor Statistics
Wage Surveys

The BLS *Industry Wage Surveys* include proprietary and nonprofit hospitals and state and local government hospitals in some of the largest Standard Metropolitan Statistical Areas (SMSAs). The exact number of SMSAs surveyed varies from year to year, although major SMSAs have been included in every survey. Since we have included all SMSAs for which wage data are presented in BLS reports in our regressions, the sample is not necessarily the same in any given year. However, to limit our analysis to the SMSAs surveyed every year would reduce our sample unnecessarily. A cost of our approach is that dynamic wage-setting equations cannot be estimated. A list of the SMSAs is presented in appendix D.

Data on both wages and fringe benefits are collected by the BLS, but we only analyze wages because it is difficult to convert fringe benefits into monetary terms. From 1966 to 1975 (in four surveys), the BLS collected data on the extent of hospital unionization by labor category, SMSA, and hospital ownership (private versus government). Union activity in hospitals before 1966 was very limited (Miller and Shortell 1969). Since gauging the impact of unionization on wages is a major objective of this study—and the impact may differ according to whether the hospital is operated privately or by government—we have included two observations for each SMSA. However, as the two types of hospitals have most explanatory variables in common, there is some question about the number of degrees of freedom applicable for hypothesis testing. We base our statistical tests on the total number of observations, but are conservative in using two-tail tests in cases when one-tail tests may well apply. As the data base is constructed, there are three hundred observations; but individual regressions contain far fewer observations because much of the analysis is based on a 1966-1975 subsample, and because of missing data.

BLS surveys are conducted by personal interview. Occupational classification is based on a uniform set of job descriptions designed to take account of interhospital and interarea variations in job content within the same job category. Apprentices and other learners are excluded; supervisors are only included in job categories specifically designated as supervisory positions.[4]

Empirical Specification

Dependent Variables and Choice of Labor Categories

The occupational categories selected for empirical analysis represent the entire spectrum of skills of hospital employees: registered nurses, licensed practical nurses, medical technologists, transcribing machine operators, switchboard operators, aides-orderlies, and porters-maids.

Registered nurses and medical technologists are professional workers. Although their skills are useful to health-related employers other than hospitals, they are unlikely to seek employment outside their professions and thus are relatively insulated from labor market conditions in the economy as a whole. Of the two occupations, the registered nurse is far more homogenous. Even though there is considerable variation among RNs in terms of educational preparation, the fact that licensure is universal provides reasonable assurance that non-RNs will not be designated RNs. Medical technologists are licensed in a few states, and national certifying bodies do exist.[5] But nonlicensed and/or noncertified technologists with comparatively little formal training and/or experience are likely to be lumped together with some highly qualified laboratory personnel, many of whom hold a baccalaureate degree. Hospitals are major employers of RNs and technologists, and, at least for RNs, market conditions within the hospital sector are thought by many to be the dominant force in wage setting.[6]

Licensed practical nurses are classified by the U.S. Census as service workers rather than as professionals. The LPN's training is shorter than either the RN's or the medical technologist's, comprising usually twelve to eighteen months. They are licensed in all states. Given their industry-specific skills, they, too, are likely to confine their job search to hospitals and related settings. Nursing aides and orderlies receive no formal preparation other than on-the-job training provided by hospitals and clinics. These individuals are neither licensed nor certified; nor is there any professional association to represent their collective interests.[7] Mobility of such persons in and out of health-related industries is much more common than it is for the other three occupational groups.

Transcribing machine and switchboard operators represent, respectively, relatively skilled and somewhat less-skilled clerical occupations. All training is on-the-job. Porters and maids are unskilled and have low status.

With the exception of the porters-maids category, for which wage rates are in hourly terms, all wage dependent variables refer to weekly wages. It would have been desirable to develop a more comprehensive wage measure incorporating the monetary value of fringe benefits. Unfortunately, however, although the BLS collects and publishes some data (for example, vacation days, types of insurance plans offered), no summary information on fringes is available. Omission of these data is particularly regrettable in assessing the impact of unions, because collective bargaining may have a greater effect on fringe benefits than on wages. All monetarily expressed variables in this study are deflated by an area price index, which varies both geographically and over time.[8]

Undeflated and deflated wage series, based on the *Industry Wage Surveys,* are presented for the seven occupations in table 3-1. Several trends are evident from the table. First, in terms of real wages, 1972 rather than 1975 was the peak year in all but one of the seven occupations, transcribing machine operators. Real wage growth prior to 1972, especially during 1963-1972, was dramatic. As a rule, the percentage growth in real wages was higher between 1963 and 1966 (that is, before the introduction of Medicare and Medicaid) than between 1966 and 1969—the first years of the Medicare-Medicaid period (rates not shown). The upward spurt in real wages clearly predated Medicare and Medicaid; these programs could nevertheless lend support to this upward trend. Second, wages increased the most in the two nursing and the porters-maids occupations; wages of transcribing machine and switchboard operators rose the least. No patterns in skill differentials are evident from table 3-1. Third, although government hospital wages remained higher than wages in private hospitals throughout the period, with the notable exception of LPNs, the differential narrowed in all but one case (transcribing machine operators, for which private wages were slightly higher in the base year).

Explanatory Variables on the Supply Side

General Labor Market Conditions. Hospitals face some competition for labor from employers in other industries.[9] Considering the occupations selected for our analysis, it is plausible that transcribing machine and switchboard operators, aides-orderlies, and porters-maids are sensitive to labor market conditions in the economy at large as well as to those within the hospital sector. Therefore in wage regressions for these four occupations we have included occupation-specific wage measures (AWAGE) from the Bureau of Labor Statistics' *Area Wage Surveys* as explanatory variables. Like the dependent variables, AWAGE is defined for SMSAs. Economy-wide wage rates for transcribing machine operators, switchboard operators, and porters-maids are available. For purposes of our aides-orderlies regressions, we have used the porters-maids series. Although aides and orderlies acquire health-care-related skills on the job, they too belong to the pool of unskilled labor force participants. We expect that in response to increases in AWAGE, hospital wages in the corresponding occupation should rise.

Wage regressions for these four occupations also include the SMSA unemployment rate (UN). To the extent that high area unemployment reflects a loose labor market, unemployment should have a negative impact on hospital wages. However, a positive association between area unemployment and wages has also been explained (see Rosen, mimeo). In areas in which employment is cyclically sensitive and therefore average unemployment is relatively high, employers must offer higher wages to compensate for the additional risk to workers. But because hospital employment is relatively immune to business cycle conditions, this argument does not apply in our context.

Several previous studies have examined the link between general labor market conditions and hospital workers' wages. Using state data, Davis (1973) estimated hospital wage regressions containing the mean manufacturing wage as an explanatory variable. Not surprisingly, the manufacturing wage parameter estimates were uniformly positive and almost always statistically significant at conventional levels. Her wage variables on both sides of her regressions refer to all occupations. Associated elasticities were in the 0.2 to 0.4 range.

Table 3-1
Trends in Hospital Wages, 1960-1975

Category	1960	1963	1966	1969	1972	1975	Growth (%)
Professional Nurses							
All undeflated	$ 79.22	$ 89.66	$107.29	$145.90	$183.56	$224.80	183.8
All deflated	109.67	112.22	136.65	165.69	182.30	176.19	60.7
Government undeflated	81.40	92.84	111.06	148.16	187.44	228.29	180.5
Government deflated	112.60	116.37	141.50	168.07	186.17	178.90	58.9
Private undeflated	77.04	86.46	103.53	143.65	179.67	222.25	188.5
Private deflated	106.74	108.07	131.80	163.13	178.43	173.74	62.8
Licensed Practical Nurses							
All undeflated	60.25	67.85	79.07	107.12	137.92	168.72	180.0
All deflated	83.10	85.02	100.43	121.43	136.72	132.21	59.1
Government undeflated	64.16	75.35	85.49	100.43	129.24	164.64	156.6
Government deflated	88.52	90.55	104.24	126.32	141.51	133.27	50.6
Private undeflated	56.24	63.68	76.00	102.76	133.12	167.65	198.1
Private deflated	77.69	79.48	96.61	116.53	131.92	130.99	68.6
Medical Technologists							
All undeflated	85.78	97.12	114.92	148.56	186.35	231.65	170.1
All deflated	188.78	121.16	146.06	168.63	184.93	181.40	52.7
Government undeflated	87.80	100.46	119.72	150.98	190.75	237.19	170.1
Government deflated	121.56	125.38	152.10	171.26	189.37	185.73	52.8
Private undeflated	83.77	93.78	110.12	146.14	181.95	227.34	171.4
Private deflated	116.01	116.93	140.02	166.00	180.49	177.52	53.0

Transcribing Machine Operators							
All undeflated	64.70	73.50	83.40	100.02	127.81	163.47	152.7
All deflated	89.44	90.70	105.96	113.52	126.80	127.73	42.8
Government undeflated	64.16	75.35	85.49	100.43	129.24	164.64	156.6
Government deflated	88.64	93.20	108.56	113.96	128.16	128.69	45.2
Private undeflated	65.25	71.65	81.30	99.62	126.38	162.47	149.0
Private deflated	90.23	88.21	103.35	113.08	125.43	126.58	40.3
Switchboard Operators							
All undeflated	60.82	66.75	75.81	91.07	117.17	147.95	143.3
All deflated	83.93	83.35	96.15	103.13	116.17	115.74	37.9
Government undeflated	65.57	70.79	80.09	94.48	121.02	151.76	131.4
Government deflated	90.43	88.55	101.56	106.96	120.09	118.81	31.4
Private undeflated	46.31	49.82	60.99	77.93	104.86	135.95	193.6
Private deflated	63.77	65.32	77.35	88.27	103.76	105.94	66.1
Porters-Maids (Hourly)							
All undeflated	1.23	1.39	1.64	2.03	2.86	3.46	181.3
All deflated	1.09	1.73	2.08	2.29	2.82	2.70	59.8
Government undeflated	1.38	1.53	1.79	2.16	2.99	3.63	163.0
Government deflated	1.89	1.92	2.26	2.44	2.94	2.83	49.7
Private undeflated	1.09	1.17	1.49	1.89	2.68	3.31	203.7
Private deflated	1.49	1.53	1.88	2.14	2.66	2.58	73.2

Source: Based on *Industry Wage Surveys: Hospitals*, Bureau of Labor Statistics.
Note: The area price index, used for deflating wage series, is expressed in 1972 dollars (1972 = 1.00). See appendix A.

In a time series, cross-sectional analysis of nonprofessional hospital workers' wages over the years 1963-1972, Salkever (1975) stressed factors related to a tightening labor market and rising welfare payments during the 1960s as hospital wage determinants. He included measures of area unemployment and Aid to Families with Dependent Children payments as explanatory variables. Although the welfare variable's coefficient was positive as anticipated, so were his coefficients on unemployment—a surprising result.

Feldstein (1971) and Feldstein and Taylor (1977) documented the rapid rise in hospital wages during the 1960s and early 1970s and emphasized the finding that, in some cities and for some occupations, hospital employees earned more than their counterparts in other sectors in the early 1970s. Our study covers more recent years and a somewhat longer time period. Considering the occupations included in our regressions for which comparable nonhospital wages have been coded, we find that as of 1975, transcribing machine and switchboard operators earned slightly more in hospitals than elsewhere, while the opposite was true of porters and maids.

Minimum Wages. An amendment to the Federal Fair Labor Standards Act, which became effective in 1967, extended federal minimum wage coverage to hospital employees. Prior to 1967, many hospital employees were covered by state minimum wage laws, the majority of which were first enacted during the 1950s and early 1960s.[10] In 1960, fourteen of the twenty-two SMSAs for which hospital wage data are generally available from the BLS had minimum wage laws;[11] of the fourteen, three exempted hospital employees.

Our minimum wage variable MWAGE equals one if a minimum wage covered hospital employees in the city and year, and equals zero otherwise. MWAGE is the higher of the federal and state mandated minimum. With a few exceptions, the federal minimum is higher.

Theoretically, statutory minimum wages should raise the wage rates of covered workers and *may* lower them for their noncovered counterparts. The word *may* is emphasized because, as Welch (1974) noted, the wage effect on noncovered persons depends on, among other factors, the elasticity of labor supply. With an infinitely elastic supply curve, noncovered workers would withdraw from the labor force until noncovered wage rates reached the statutory minimum. An empirical isue concerns compliance. If employers disobey the law and/or employees fear to complain about subminimum wages lest they lose their jobs, the effects of minimum wage laws on both covered and noncovered workers' wages will be small. According to Gramlich (1976), compliance with minimum wage legislation has been far from complete. However, there is some empirical evidence that minimum wages raise area wages for covered and noncovered workers taken together (Cotterill and Wadycki 1976), and those for covered workers in particular (Katz 1973). To our knowledge, only Taylor (1977) has assessed the effects of minimum wage coverage in a hospital context, evaluating its impact on hospital demand for labor. Of course, the effects of minimum wages on incomes, an issue *not* considered in our study, depends on employment as well as wage impacts.[12]

For conceptual reasons, it would have been desirable to develop two minimum wage variables, one for statutes covering hospital employees and another for statutes that exclude them. However, the latter situation occurred too infrequently during the study period to permit such a distinction to be made. For this reason, for observations when a state statute excluded hospital employees, MWAGE takes the value zero.

Comparisons between the actual mean wage for an occupation and the minimum wage have often led to the misleading inference that if the former exceeds the latter, the minimum wage can have no effect. It is quite possible, however, that hospitals (and other employers) seek to maintain a wage hierarchy within their organizations. Hence, if wages in low skilled occupations increase, so will those for more highly skilled employees.[13] We include MWAGE as an explanatory variable in wage regressions for all seven occupations.

Unionization. With the extension of the National Labor Relations Act to employees of nonprofit hospitals in 1974, it is reasonable to expect a substantial and continuing growth in unionization activity in hospitals. Conditional forecasts of the effects of unions on hospital wages in particular, and costs in general, are thus of considerable public policy as well as scholarly interest. Before presenting our specification of the union component, it is useful to review past research on union effects in a hospital context. The literature on unions in other sectors is far too voluminous for us to consider here.

Feldman and Scheffler (1977) estimated the effects of unions on four classes of hospital employees: RNs, LPNs, general secretaries, and housekeeping employees. Their regression analysis was principally based on data from the University of North Carolina's 1977 Survey of Hospital Labor Markets. The survey provided information on wages and union coverage for employees in each of the four labor categories, including such factors as whether there was a union election or a job action during the preceding twelve months. Information on fringe benefits was also obtained. The authors' specification was somewhat complicated by the extensive use of interaction terms, making the empirical results difficult to interpret. Results were presented by occupation. Union wage effects ranged from 3.4 to 11.8 percent; they were highest for secretaries and lowest for RNs. The authors presented what they called "tentative" results on the union effect on fringe benefits.[14] Evaluated at the variables' means, unionization increased the monetary value of fringe benefits about 6 percent.

Sloan and Elnicki (1978) estimated a wage equation for RNs containing a dummy variable equal to one if the hospital had a collective bargaining unit covering RNs. The principal data source was the Survey of Hospital Directors of Nursing conducted at the University of Florida during 1973. Twelve percent of hospital respondents had collective bargaining agreements covering RNs (no other measures of union activity were obtained). Sloan and Elnicki found union effects on wages from 0 to 4 percent, the latter figure being essentially the same as the Feldman-Scheffler estimate for RNs. They then considered the possibility that unionization is endogenous and estimated a two-equation model with RN wages and collective bargaining of RNs as the dependent variables and two-stage least squares as the estimator.[15] Using this approach, a zero union effect on wages was obtained.

A study by Link and Landon (1975) of RN wages, based on the authors' own 1973 survey of RN wages and unionization, used a somewhat different measure—the percentage of nurses in a hospital covered by collective bargaining agreements. In hospitals in which at least 75 percent of nurses are covered, the authors estimated that annual starting salaries of baccalaureate and diploma nurses rise by $500 to $800 (in 1973 dollars), or from 5 to 10 percent, compared to hospitals with no union coverage.

Fottler (1977) examined the impact of unions on wages of nonprofessional hospital employees. Fottler used BLS data on hospital wages and unions, which we also use in this chapter; but his time period was shorter (1966-1972) than ours, and this limited the number of explanatory variables that could be included. Perhaps his most interesting result in the present context was the finding of a statistically significant, positive union impact on wages of between 4.5 and 8.2 percent, on average. Fottler estimated this impact to be on the order of 1 to 2 percent on total hospital costs, which was interpreted as being relatively unimportant to the inflationary trend during the 1966-1972 period. However, his assessment did not include nonwage influences of unionization, such as on staffing, labor/nonlabor substitution, and turnover.

Davis' (1973) analysis of average wage rates in community hospitals, based on American Hospital Association (AHA) surveys, included two measures of the threat of unionization, but no measures of union coverage itself. The two measures were the percent of nonagricultural workers belonging to a union in the state, and a binary variable taking the value one if the state had a law requiring voluntary hospitals to recognize a union when so requested by the majority of employees of a bargaining unit. The coefficients of the first threat variable were generally insignificant with an unanticipated negative sign. Coefficients of the second were generally positive and significant.[16] Feldman and Scheffler (1977) also evaluated threat effects. Their variable, reflecting the percent of *hospitals* (as opposed to nonagricultural workers) in a state with collective bargaining, showed no effect, but a threat effect *within* the hospital was detected. Specifically, secretaries' wages were 9 percent higher if another occupation within the hospital was organized.

Miller, Becker, and Krinsky (1977) have described a comprehensive evaluation of hospital union effects in three states: Minnesota, Illinois, and Wisconsin. Data were obtained by mailed questionnaire. Unfortunately, the authors reported only their findings without displaying their methodology or presenting detailed tables. Hence, we are unable to evaluate the results they obtained, which are as follows: First, on average, unions raised relative occupational wages about 5 percent and fringe benefits by 8.4 percent. Second, unionized hospitals experienced approximately 5 percent higher costs from the union effect on grievance procedures, personnel practices, and the like. Yet, third, employee turnover was 50 percent lower in unionized hospitals; and the authors estimated this factor alone resulted in savings in average (labor and nonlabor) costs of about 2 to 4 percent. The author found that the first two factors offset the third. They concluded that the net effect of unions was to raise average costs 2 to 4 percent, a level which suggested (to the authors) that ". . . unions are probably not going to be a major source of inflation in the near future"(p. 517).

In another study (Sloan and Steinwald, forthcoming, 1980), we found that unions have had much larger positive impacts on average labor and average labor plus nonlabor costs in hospitals. To illustrate, the union impacts on average labor cost per patient day were in the 2 to 14 percent range. Moreover, Elnicki (1975) could not detect a tendency for unionization of professional nurses in hospitals to reduce nurse turnover, let alone a 50 percent reduction. Of course, Elnicki's study dealt only with nurses, while the Miller et al. evaluation included other personnel as well.

We turn now to our union variable (UNION). Every three years from 1966 through 1975, the BLS has published estimates of the percentage of hospitals in selected SMSAs having collective bargaining agreements covering a *majority* of their employees. Except in 1975, the BLS provided separate estimates for RNs, other professional and technical, office-clerical, and other nonprofessional employees, with each being available for both nongovernment (primarily nonprofit) and state and local governmental hospitals. In 1975, the first two and the latter two occupational groups were combined into professional-technical and nonprofessional categories, respectively.

So as not to lose the detail available in earlier years in constructing our union variable, we have assumed that the *ratio* of RN coverage to that of other professional and technical employees in the SMSA was the same in 1975 as in 1972. The same assumption was used for nonprofessional employees. The seven occupations have been matched with the four union categories. For example, aides-orderlies and porters-maids fall into the nonprofessional employees' union classification. Considering all the years included in our empirical analysis of union impacts, 1966-1975, the nonprofessional category has been the most unionized (mean of UNION = 32.1 percent), followed by RNs (21.0 percent), office clerical (19.2 percent), and other professional (14.2 percent).

In general, UNION takes higher values for state and local government than for private hospitals. To ascertain whether unions in government hospitals have differential wage impacts (as compared to unions in private hospitals), some regressions contain the variable GUNION, which is UNION multiplied by a binary variable G, which is one for government hospitals. A regression presented in appendix C shows that the extent of hospital unionization in the SMSA, not surprisingly, is strongly associated with unionization of nonagricultural employees in the state in which the SMSA is located. For theoretical reasons and from previous empirical research, the anticipated signs of the UNION coefficients are positive. In this instance in particular, we are not only interested in hypothesis testing regarding the direction of effect, but also in gauging the magnitude of the wage response to collective bargaining activity.

Licensure. Licensure of certain occupations is justified to the public as a means to protect ignorant consumers against unscrupulous and incompetent providers; but it is frequently argued, with some empirical support, that licensure also benefits the occupational groups fortunate enough to obtain the franchise. As already noted, nursing associations have successfully fought for mandatory licensure, which presumably protects nurses better than permissive licensure. As of 1960, twelve of the twenty-two SMSAs for which the BLS generally presents hospital wage data had mandatory licensure for RNs,[17] while only eight required licensing of LPNs.[18] By 1975, licensure of RNs and LPNs was still permissive in just two of the SMSAs. By the same year, medical technologists were licensed in only four of the BLS cities. The variable MLC equals one if the state has mandatory licensure in the case of RNs and LPNs. For medical technologists, MLC equals one for any kind of licensure, as the number of states with medical technologist licensure is insufficient to maintain the mandatory-permissive distinction. We hypothesize that MLC has positive impacts on wages.

Manpower Training. Between 1961 and 1974, the number of RN graduates grew by 123 percent; the rise in LPN graduates from 1962 to 1974 was 153 percent.[19] One may reasonably expect that these dramatic increases should have negative (partial) impacts on wages in these occupations. Sloan and Elnicki (1978) found a negative relationship for RNs. Variables RNGRAD, LPNGRAD, and TCGRAD represent the number of graduates of professional nursing, practical nursing, and medical technology programs per 1,000 population in the states in which our SMSAs are located.

Locational Amenities. In equilibrium, higher real wages are paid to compensate persons willing to work (and live) in less-desirable settings. A comprehensive list of locational amenities would include cultural and recreational opportunities, pleasant climate, good schools, a clean environment, and a low crime rate. Summary "quality of life" indexes have been developed recently that collapse the many dimensions of living in a location into a few variables.[20] However, these indexes are not available as a time series of cross sections that can be matched with the communities available from the BLS. As an alternative, we have included two variables, homicides (MUR) and auto thefts (AUTO) per

100,000 population in the state in which the SMSA is located. The homicide rate reflects crimes against persons; the auto theft rate is a relatively well-measured indicator of property crimes. As defined, both MUR and AUTO are hypothesized to have positive impacts on the dependent wage variables. These variables only enter the nursing and technologist regressions.

Monopsony. Numerous studies have assessed the impact of monopsony on wage levels, both for nonhealth occupations (for example, Landon 1970, and Landon and Baird 1971) and for nursing. That some skilled health occupations are probably subject to a degree of monopsonistic exploitation by employers makes a certain amount of sense. First, there are frequently few hospitals, often only one, in a locality.[21] Second, many persons with health-specific skills are "secondary" wage earners, which limits their geographic mobility. Given their skills, there may be few, if any, alternative employers in the locality. This limitation, of course, would not exist for unskilled and/or semiskilled nonhospital-specific labor. Third, there is some anecdotal evidence that hospitals in some larger cities set wages and other conditions of employment in concert (see Yett 1970). In single hospital communities, the hospital is potentially a natural monopsonist. By contrast, in multihospital areas, there must be collusion among hospitals.

Since direct evidence of collusion is generally lacking, it is standard practice among economists to assume that the costs of colluding are directly related to the degree of hospital concentration. Hurd (1973) and Fottler (1977) gauged concentration by the percentage of total hospital employment in a given city accounted for by the eight largest hospitals. Both Davis (1973) and Taylor (1977) included bed/population ratios as measures of hospital density. The most concerted efforts to measure hospital concentration to date are studies by Link and Landon (1975 and 1976). These authors constructed three measures of concentration: a four-firm concentration ratio, defined in a manner similar to Hurd's and Fottler's eight-firm measure; a Herfindahl index, calculated by summing the squares of each firm's percentage share of total beds in the city; and an entropy index, $E = S_1 \log S_1 + S_2 \log S_1 \ldots + S_n \log S_n$, where E is the concentration measure, and S is the hospital's share of total beds in the city.

Although these studies have found empirical support for the notion that hospitals exercise monopsony power in the market for professional nursing services, there is reason to question the validity of their empirical tests. We present our four measures of hospital concentration in appendix D: four- and eight-firm, Herfindahl, and entropy indexes. It is quite apparent from our data that concentration, irrespective of the measure employed, varies inversely with city size. In all of the studies previously cited, the wage dependent variables appear to be in nominal rather than real terms. The negative signs on the concentration variables in the wage regressions are consistent with the view that, rather than capturing monopsony influences, these estimated coefficients are only confirming a well-known fact: cost of living, other things being equal, is higher in large cities. Consequently, in equilibrium, nominal wages are also comparatively high in large cities. Until more direct measures of monopsony power can be constructed, it seems wise to postpone empirical tests of the monopsony hypothesis. No monopsony variable is included in our wage regressions.

Explanatory Variables on the Demand Side

As we discussed in chapter 2, in a competitive labor market, variables expressing geographic and temporal variations in product demand will have no effect on real wages in equilibrium, unless the long-run labor supply curve is upward-sloping, as may be the case with heterogeneous (employee) tastes. Until the market clears, variables accounting for demand curve shifts will affect wages even if the long-run labor supply curve is horizontal. If the labor market contains monopsonistic elements, demand-shift variables affect wages, even in equilibrium.

Income. The variable INC is per capita income in the SMSA, deflated by an area price index. It is expected to have a positive impact on wages—if, in fact, it has an impact. Unemployment, classified as a supply-side variable, could, like income, be construed as a demand-side variable as well.

Third-Party Reimbursement. In research on hospital behavior, substantial policy interest has centered around the impact of third-party reimbursement. During the period covered by our study, the major health policy event was the introduction of Medicare and Medicaid during the mid-1960s. An important issue in this and later chapters concerns the degree to which the ensuing infusion of government funds has boosted both hospital wage rates and wage bills.

The variable REIM is the fraction of hospital expense covered by private *and* public insurance in the state in which the SMSA is located. The variable has been constructed from AHA data on hospital expenses and third-party payments from private and government sources. Unfortunately, the latter data are not available for SMSAs. Since information on private insurance payments to hospitals is unavailable on a state basis, we have been forced to take national estimates of the proportion of total Blue Cross and commercial insurance payments going to hospitals (which are available by year) and apply these proportions to state data on total Blue Cross and commercial payments for all health services.

Physician Availability. Several empirical studies of hospital behavior contain measures of physician availability.[22] Consumers demand health care services from doctors who in turn select inputs, including hospital services. For this reason, and because they tend to hospitalize patients in the vicinity of their offices, demand for hospital services should be higher where doctors are located. The variable MD is the number of nonfederal, office-based physicians per 1,000 population in the SMSA.[23]

Hospital Bed Availability. According to "Roemer's law," the supply of beds generates its own demand.[24] This notion has been debated and evaluated for years,[25] but few would contend that area bed supply has no impact on hospital utilization. Our measure BEDS is the number of nonfederal, short-term general hospital beds per 1,000 population in the SMSA.

Standardizing Variables. Even a casual examination of the BLS hospital wage levels and trends (see table 3-1) indicates that government hospitals generally pay higher wages than nongovernment hospitals, although the differences have generally been declining over time. Perhaps government hospitals, holding such factors as unionization constant, are less-desirable places to work on the whole. Alternatively, this could be a disequilibrium differential that will disappear over time. Variables G and GTA are, respectively, a binary variable identifying government hospital observations and an interaction between G and a time trend, with 1960 equal to 1.

Empirical Results

Overview

The functional form in all of this chapter's regressions is linear. Regressions in tables 3-2 and 3-3 are based on data from 1960 through 1975; tables 3-4 and 3-5 on data from 1966 through 1975. The principal difference between the two sets of regressions is that the latter contains estimates of union impacts. As noted earlier, data on hospital unions are only available from 1966 on. The even-numbered tables contain nursing and medical technologist regressions; the odd-numbered ones present empirical results for the two office-clerical occupations, as well as the for aides-orderlies and porters-maids categories.

Viewing these tables overall, it is not possible to state that either demand- or supply-side variables dominate. A number of both types are statistically significant at conventional levels, and yet there are also some disappointing results for both types. F-statistics on the regressions are uniformly significant at the 1 percent level. R^2s vary from around 0.3 to 0.6, which is respectable for a time series of cross sections. Our discussion of results on individual explanatory variables follows the order used in the specification section.

Table 3-2
Wage Regressions for Nursing Occupations and Medical Technologists, 1960-1975

Occupation	CONS	G	GTA	MWAGE	RNGRAD	LPNGRAD	REIM	INC	MD	BEDS	MLC	MUR	AUTO	
							Explanatory Variables							
Professional nurses	139.30	-27.73* (8.31)	2.90* (0.67)	18.73* (3.06)	-12.77 (15.39)									$R^2 = 0.41$ $F(4,143) = 24.7$
Professional nurses	52.37	-11.20 (7.87)	1.49* (0.64)	12.99* (2.96)	-20.67 (17.82)		2.54 (17.44)	0.026* (0.0042)	-4.59 (6.25)	-2.18 (2.92)	6.06 (4.97)			$R^2 = 0.55$ $F(9,138) = 18.7$
Professional nurses	57.31	-3.85 (7.40)	0.86 (0.60)	11.44* (2.74)	-1.92 (17.83)		5.28 (15.96)	0.017* (0.0042)	0.11 (6.04)	-2.62 (2.69)	8.47*** (4.57)	1.36* (0.28)	0.0072 (0.0053)	$R^2 = 0.63$ $F(11,136) = 21.1$
Licensed practical nurses	95.54	-16.42** (7.53)	1.96* (0.61)	18.80* (2.83)		-12.22 (24.20)								$R^2 = 0.40$ $F(4,145) = 23.7$
Licensed practical nurses	22.42	-2.62 (7.39)	0.77 (0.60)	13.00* (2.85)		-8.69 (26.29)	27.11*** (14.46)	0.017* (0.0038)	-8.38 (5.37)	-1.85 (5.37)	11.19* (2.11)			$R^2 = 0.52$ $F(9,140) = 17.1$
Licensed practical nurses	23.75	-1.20 (7.41)	0.65 (0.60)	12.03* (2.89)		-1.81 (26.45)	30.74** (15.03)	0.013* (0.0043)	-6.95 (5.59)	-1.04 (2.17)	9.42* (3.13)	0.39 (0.27)	0.0065 (0.0053)	$R^2 = 0.51$ $F(11,138) = 13.1$
Medical technologists	142.57	-19.44** (9.73)	2.44** (0.78)	17.17* (3.67)										$R^2 = 0.29$ $F(3,146) = 20.0$
Medical technologists	-0.35	2.15 (8.91)	0.59 (0.72)	4.81 (3.54)			31.45*** (16.84)	0.031* (0.0047)	-1.97 (6.75)	2.26 (2.52)	23.10* (4.15)			$R^2 = 0.52$ $F(8,141) = 19.3$
Medical technologists	0.54	2.55 (9.04)	0.56 (0.73)	4.78 (3.60)			32.54*** (17.83)	0.029* (0.0054)	-1.03 (7.45)	2.36 (2.57)	22.31* (4.54)	0.14 (0.35)	0.0011 (0.0064)	$R^2 = 0.52$ $F(10,139) = 15.2$

Note: Figures in parentheses are standard errors.
*Significant at 1 percent level (two-tail test); **Significant at 5 percent level (two-tail test); ***Significant at 10 percent level (two-tail test).

Table 3-3
Wage Regressions for Office-Clerical Occupations, Aides-Orderlies, and Porters-Maids, 1960-1975

Occupation	CONS	G	GTA	AWAGE[a]	MWAGE	REIM	INC	MD	BEDS	UN	
Transcribing machine operators	63.92	-14.59* (5.44)	1.54* (0.44)	0.38* (0.12)	8.08* (2.10)						$R^2 = 0.36$ $F(4,139) = 19.8$
Transcribing machine operators	29.17	-5.65 (5.42)	0.77*** (0.44)	0.13 (0.13)	5.48* (2.08)	9.56 (10.47)	0.014* (0.003)	6.04 (3.94)	-0.99 (1.54)		$R^2 = 0.48$ $F(8,135) = 15.4$
Switchboard operators	31.50	1.74 (5.07)	0.62 (0.42)	0.60* (0.12)	6.75* (1.95)					2.16 (8.97)	$R^2 = 0.47$ $F(5,136) = 24.5$
Switchboard operators	-13.00	5.72 (4.74)	0.26 (0.39)	0.10 (0.15)	4.76** (1.80)	41.49* (10.57)	0.012* (0.003)	8.80* (3.38)	2.12 (1.38)	-4.57 (8.53)	$R^2 = 0.60$ $F(9,132) = 21.6$
Aides-orderlies	48.48	-17.67* (6.30)	2.28* (0.51)	11.18* (2.59)	11.31* (2.42)					0.13 (11.95)	$R^2 = 0.45$ $F(5,138) = 22.3$
Aides-orderlies	-26.41	-5.89 (6.45)	1.26** (0.53)	5.24*** (2.97)	6.93* (2.45)	32.95** (15.01)	0.011* (0.003)	13.14* (4.44)	3.01*** (1.81)	-4.49 (11.68)	$R^2 = 0.54$ $F(9,134) = 17.7$
Porters-maids[b]	0.68	-0.19 (0.17)	0.0043* (0.0014)	0.45* (0.07)	0.30* (0.07)					0.22 (0.33)	$R^2 = 0.48$ $F(5,132) = 24.5$
Porters-maids[b]	-1.56	0.15 (0.17)	0.0013 (0.0015)	0.27* (0.08)	0.17* (0.07)	1.09* (0.41)	0.00027* (0.00009)	0.23*** (0.12)	0.17* (0.05)	-0.003 (0.32)	$R^2 = 0.57$ $F(9,128) = 19.1$

Note: Figures in parentheses are standard errors.

*Significant at the 1 percent level (two-tail test); **Significant at the 5 percent level (two-tail test); ***Significant at the 10 percent level (two-tail test).

[a]AWAGE is in weekly terms for transcribing machine and switchboard operators, and in hourly terms for the rest.

[b]Dependent variable is in hourly terms.

Table 3-4
Wage Regressions for Nursing Occupations and Medical Technologists, 1966-1975

Occupation	CONS	G	MWAGE	RNGRAD	LPNGRAD	TCGRAD	UNION
			Explanatory Variables				
Professional nurses	134.21	5.15 (3.50)	20.81* (3.70)	−8.03 (18.61)			12.19** (5.90)
Professional nurses	2.53	5.72** (2.82)	10.65* (3.35)	4.64 (20.62)			8.16*** (5.08)
Professional nurses	38.27	5.23** (2.62)	9.78* (3.13)	2.30 (19.96)			11.01** (4.78)
Professional nurses	36.71	8.34* (3.03)	9.68* (3.09)	7.76 (19.88)			24.67* (8.39)
Licensed practical nurses	88.95	2.22 (2.99)	18.00* (3.25)		19.30 (26.39)		26.50* (6.06)
Licensed practical nurses	15.24	2.49 (2.70)	13.27* (3.40)		−30.25 (33.73)		20.56* (5.92)
Licensed practical nurses	25.59	2.60 (2.70)	12.54* (3.43)		−28.29 (33.66)		19.85* (5.93)
Licensed practical nurses	34.84	5.14*** (2.88)	13.45* (3.39)		−30.42 (33.10)		56.62* (17.49)
Medical technologists	130.34	3.90 (3.97)	14.99* (4.09)			57.18* (22.09)	38.85* (8.08)
Medical technologists	7.38	6.06** (3.21)	3.45 (3.73)			48.76** (20.47)	20.26* (7.19)
Medical technologists	−3.43	6.10*** (3.23)	3.60 (3.78)			55.8* (21.6)	20.46* (7.23)
Medical technologists	1.29	7.27* (3.51)	4.00 (3.81)			56.60* (21.64)	37.69*** (21.49)

Note: Figures in parentheses are standard errors.

*Significant at 1 percent level (two-tail test); **Significant at 5 percent level (two-tail test); ***Significant at 10 percent level (two-tail test).

Supply-Side Results

The first variables on the supply side, alternative wages outside the hospital (AWAGE) and area unemployment (UN), are only included in table 3-3 and table 3-5 regressions. Somewhat surprisingly, AWAGE by no means dominates these regressions. In fact, in variants containing the full specification, the parameter on AWAGE is sometimes negative. When positive *and* statistically significant, the marginal effect of a dollar increase in AWAGE on the hospital wage is always far less than unity.[26] Taken together, the results on AWAGE suggest any or all of the following: First, occupations with a common title may be heterogeneous across industries and hence noncompeting. Second, there may be segmented labor markets; wage differentials for a given type of work do not disappear because workers may be immobile among industries. Third, there may be a disequilibrium, which is either temporary or permanent (because of a

GUNION	REIM	INC	MD	BEDS	MLC	MUR	AUTO	
								$R^2 = 0.29$ $F(4,111) = 11.2$
	23.05 (19.25)	0.035* (0.0045)	2.90 (6.94)	−4.91 (3.29)	2.11 (5.08)			$R^2 = 0.56$ $F(9,106) = 15.0$
	7.92 (18.15)	0.023* (0.005)	3.01 (6.62)	−4.18 (3.09)	6.54 (4.84)	1.37* (0.32)	0.0073 (0.0057)	$R^2 = 0.63$ $F(11,104) = 16.1$
−18.68** (9.49)	11.53 (18.00)	0.022* (0.0049)	1.62 (6.57)	−4.86 (3.07)	6.74 (4.78)	1.47* (0.33)	0.0070 (0.0056)	$R^2 = 0.64$ $F(12,103) = 15.5$
								$R^2 = 0.39$ $F(4,119) = 19.0$
	17.72 (18.71)	0.023* (0.0046)	−8.74 (6.27)	−2.86 (2.22)	7.83** (3.28)			$R^2 = 0.53$ $F(9,114) = 14.4$
	13.88 (18.97)	0.019* (0.0059)	−9.02 (6.48)	−2.50 (2.31)	6.72** (3.35)	0.22 (0.31)	0.0080 (0.0055)	$R^2 = 0.54$ $F(11,112) = 12.1$
−39.44** (17.69)	10.37 (18.71)	0.018* (0.0054)	−13.74** (6.71)	−2.65 (2.28)	6.95** (3.29)	0.22 (0.31)	0.0071 (0.0053)	$R^2 = 0.56$ $F(12,111) = 11.9$
								$R^2 = 0.34$ $F(4,119) = 15.7$
	38.17*** (19.71)	0.032* (0.005)	−2.28 (7.54)	−1.45 (2.78)	23.51* (4.95)			$R^2 = 0.60$ $F(9,114) = 19.0$
	41.65** (20.42)	0.028* (0.007)	3.04 (8.10)	−0.98 (2.83)	22.66* (5.08)	0.40 (0.40)	−0.0025 (0.0065)	$R^2 = 0.60$ $F(11,112) = 15.5$
−18.39 (21.60)	40.52** (20.49)	0.027* (0.007)	1.28 (8.37)	−1.11 (2.83)	22.38* (5.10)	0.41 (0.40)	−0.0028 (0.0065)	$R^2 = 0.61$ $F(12,111) = 14.3$

specific restraint on interindustry mobility). There is some collinearity between AWAGE and several of the other explanatory variables; for example, the area health resource-variables—physicians and hospital beds. But the correlations are not sufficiently strong to fully explain these results.

According to one standard economic argument, the area unemployment rate (UN), as a measure of market tightness, should have a negative impact on hospital wages. We always obtain negative, albeit highly insignificant, UN coefficients in table 3-5. In table 3-3, however, there are some positive signs on this variable. Coupled with our findings on AWAGE, the UN results do not support the view that general labor market conditions provide an important explanation of variations in wages of nonprofessional hospital employees.

The minimum wage variable (MWAGE) enters all regressions in the four tables. Elasticities based on some of the regressions, evaluated at the variable means, are presented in table 3-6. With one exception, the MWAGE parameter estimates are both positive and statistically significant at conventional levels. Although the associated elasticities are modest, ranging from 0.03 to 0.15, it is

Table 3-5
Wage Regressions for Office-Clerical Occupations, Aides-Orderlies, Porters-Maids, 1966-1975

Occupation	CONS	G	AWAGE[a]	MWAGE	UNION	GUNION	REIM	INC	MD	BEDS	UN	
							Explanatory Variables					
Transcribing machine operators	53.66	0.002 (2.40)	0.45* (0.13)	10.01* (2.35)	10.93** (4.23)							$R^2 = 0.32$ $F(4,117) = 13.9$
Transcribing machine operators	13.41	0.59 (2.01)	-0.003 (0.133)	5.12** (2.19)	5.86 (3.82)		21.16*** (11.52)	0.022* (0.003)	9.40* (3.79)	-4.20* (1.56)		$R^2 = 0.56$ $F(8,113) = 17.7$
Transcribing machine operators	13.03	0.78 (2.28)	-0.02 (0.14)	5.11** (2.19)	7.50 (9.98)	-1.88 (10.59)	21.30*** (11.60)	0.022* (0.003)	9.43* (3.81)	-4.19* (1.57)		$R^2 = 0.56$ $F(9,112) = 15.6$
Switchboard operators	25.10	7.38* (2.10)	0.65* (0.13)	7.53* (2.21)	9.75* (3.77)							$R^2 = 0.50$ $F(5,116) = 23.1$
Switchboard operators	-29.06	8.48* (1.88)	0.15 (0.17)	3.88*** (2.04)	4.39 (3.55)		48.86* (11.84)	0.014* (0.004)	11.40* (3.56)	0.80 (1.47)		$R^2 = 0.63$ $F(9,112) = 20.9$
Switchboard operators	-28.47	9.35* (2.10)	0.14 (0.17)	3.93*** (2.04)	12.25 (9.18)	-8.96 (9.65)	49.86* (11.90)	0.014* (0.004)	11.27* (3.57)	0.74 (1.47)	-3.82 (8.62)	$R^2 = 0.63$ $F(10,111) = 18.8$
Aides-orderlies	52.00	6.62* (2.52)	7.25* (2.82)	13.15* (2.84)	20.01* (3.92)						-1.50 (11.80)	$R^2 = 0.46$ $F(5,112) = 18.9$
Aides-orderlies	-40.34	5.86* (2.18)	0.24 (2.91)	3.82 (2.91)	17.62* (3.61)		47.66* (15.97)	0.019* (0.003)	14.08* (4.40)	-0.88 (1.89)	-0.45 (10.85)	$R^2 = 0.62$ $F(9,108) = 19.5$
Aides-orderlies	-42.04	7.25* (2.95)	-0.40 (3.05)	3.65 (2.92)	20.75* (5.75)	-4.80 (6.85)	49.71* (16.27)	0.019* (0.004)	13.74* (4.44)	-0.93 (1.90)	-0.73 (10.88)	$R^2 = 0.62$ $F(10,107) = 17.5$
Porters-maids[b]	0.81	0.26* (0.07)	0.35* (0.08)	0.33* (0.08)	0.46* (0.11)							$R^2 = 0.50$ $F(5,108) = 21.5$
Porters-maids[b]	-1.48	0.26* (0.07)	0.20** (0.09)	0.13 (0.09)	0.34* (0.11)		1.18** (0.49)	0.00034* (0.00010)	0.22*** (0.13)	0.11*** (0.06)	0.005 (0.32)	$R^2 = 0.58$ $F(9,104) = 16.3$
Porters-maids[b]	-1.48	0.26* (0.09)	0.20* (0.09)	0.13*** (0.08)	0.34** (0.17)	-0.002 (0.21)	1.18** (0.50)	0.00034* (0.00011)	0.22 (0.14)	0.11*** (0.06)	0.005 (0.33)	$R^2 = 0.58$ $F(9,104) = 14.5$

Note: Figures in parentheses are standard errors.

*Significant at the 1 percent level (two-tail test); **Significant at the 5 percent level (two-tail test); ***Significant at the 10 percent level (two-tail test).

[a]AWAGE is in weekly terms for transcribing machine and switchboard operators, and in hourly terms for the rest.

[b]Dependent variable is in hourly terms. Remaining dependent variables are weekly wages.

Table 3-6
Minimum Wage Elasticities

Occupation	Tables and Regression Number	MWAGE Coefficient	Elasticity
Professional nurses	3-2(3)	11.44	0.09
	3-4(3)	9.78	0.08
Licensed practical nurses	3-2(6)	12.03	0.14
	3-4(8)	13.45	0.15
Medical technologists	3-2(9)	4.78	0.04
	3-4(11)	3.60	0.03
Transcribing machine operators	3-3(2)	5.48	0.07
	3-5(2)	5.12	0.06
Switchboard operators	3-3(4)	4.76	0.06
	3-5(5)	3.88	0.05
Aides-orderlies	3-3(6)	6.93	0.06
	3-5(8)	3.82	0.05
Porters-maids	3-3(8)	0.17	0.10
	3-5(11)	0.13	0.07

clear from table 3-6, as well as from tables 3-2 through 3-5, which give statistical significance (in parentheses), that rising minimum wages have made some contribution to hospital wage inflation. The minimum wage has had a positive impact on wages in nursing, which are set substantially above the minimums, as well as on porters, and maids' wages, which are much more likely to be at or around the minimums. These results imply that hospitals seek to maintain a wage structure.

When the lowest wage scales rise, all scales are affected. The standard neoclassical model of labor markets predicts that wages of skilled workers rise as wages of their lower-priced substitutes rise; but, for imperfect substitutes, the increase in skilled wages in response to the minimum wage should be smaller than for those with lower skills. We find that wages in some higher skilled occupations are at least as responsive.

Estimates of the impact of unions on hospital wages are found in tables 3-4, 3-5, and 3-7. Parameter estimates on UNION are always positive and generally statistically significant. Table 3-7 shows expected increases in real hospital wages if hospitals in an SMSA went from nonunion (all hospitals having less than half of their employees in a category covered, UNION = 0) to complete union coverage (every hospital having over half of employees in a category covered, UNION = 1.0). The estimated percentage increases in wages range from 4 percent (for switchboard operators) to nearly 18 percent (for aides-orderlies). These increases are within the ranges often reported economywide (see Lewis 1963). Our estimates are somewhat higher than those obtained for nonprofessional hospital workers by Fottler (1977), who used the same definition of union coverage as we use in this chapter. The estimate of a 7.4 percent increase for RNs is higher than those reported by Feldman and Scheffler (1977), which

Table 3-7
Effects of Unions on Hospital Wages

Occupation	Table and Regression Number	UNION Coefficient	Percent Increase[a]
Professional nurses	3-4(3)	11.01	6.5
Licensed practical nurses	3-4(7)	19.85	16.1
Medical technologists	3-4(11)	20.46	11.9
Transcribing machine operators	3-5(2)	5.86	4.9
Switchboard operators	3-5(5)	4.39	4.0
Aides-orderlies	3-5(8)	17.62	17.6
Porters-maids	3-5(11)	0.34	13.6

[a](Coefficient/mean wage) × 100.

were in the 3 percent range, and by Sloan and Elnicki (1978), which went from 0 to 4 percent. Our tables clearly imply that increased hospital unionization is a force to be reckoned with, especially from the perspective of hospital cost containment. We say more on this issue in later chapters.

Several regressions include both UNION and GUNION, a specification that allows us to distinguish between the influence of unions in private and in government hospitals. Judging from the parameter estimates on the GUNION variable, the impact of unions in private hospital settings is uniformly greater. Differences are statistically significant in the cases of RNs and LPNs. With GUNION included, the UNION coefficients sometimes increase substantially, in several cases by an implausible amount.

Estimates of the effects of licensure have been obtained for the nursing occupations and medical technologists. Mandatory licensure (MLC) demonstrates positive effects on RN and LPN wages with statistically significant coefficients in some RN and all LPN regressions. For medical technologists, MLC is 1 if the state licenses persons in this occupation (we do not make the mandatory-permissive distinction); the MLC parameter estimates are always statistically significant in these regressions. The estimates for LPNs in table 3-4 imply that mandatory licensure raises real wages by 5 to 6 percent on the average. Estimates based on table 3-2 are somewhat higher than this. Effects for medical technologists, based on the MLC estimates from table 3-4, are around 13 percent. Licensure in general and mandatory licensure in particular may improve worker quality, which in turn may be reflected in higher compensation levels. On the whole, however, our results indicate one can be much more confident that licensure raises real wages of persons in covered occupations.

We included measures of output of training programs in the state in table 3-2 and 3-4 regressions (RNGRAD, LPNGRAD, TCGRAD). On the basis of theory and past empirical research, negative signs were anticipated, but in the majority of cases the parameter estimates are positive. We are unable to explain these results.

Two locational amenity variables, MUR for homicides and AUTO for auto thefts per 100,000 population, are included in some regressions for professional employees. For RNs, associated coefficients on MUR are positive and statistically significant, as anticipated. Other MUR coefficients are insignificant. The AUTO variable demonstrates no impact on wages.

Variables REIM, INC, MD, and BEDS represent potential wage determinants from the hospital product demand side. Probably the most interesting among these is third-party reimbursement (REIM), represented by the fraction of hospital costs covered by private and public insurance. Table 3-8, based on tables 3-2 through 3-5, presents elasticities associated with REIM.

Many of the REIM parameter estimates are statistically significant, a sufficient number to permit the conclusion that, on the whole, increased third-party coverage has raised real hospital wages. The elasticities are among the highest we obtain in this chapter; some approach 0.4. An exception is RNs. One would predict that the growth in private and public insurance would have its greatest impact on wages of individuals with specialized health skills. This seems to be true for medical technologists, but not for RNs.

The INC parameter estimates are statistically significant at the 1 percent level in all regressions presented in tables 3-2 through 3-5. Associated elasticities for INC parameters shown in table 3-9 vary from 0.4 to 0.8. Clearly, rising real per capita income has had an important role in the growth of real hospital wages. This factor provides a good explanation of hospital wage growth during the 1960s, especially in the years immediately preceding Medicare and Medicaid. Since 1970, real per capita income has increased relatively slowly.

Our final product demand variables pertain to physician (MD) and bed (BEDS) density. The physician-population ratio variable shows no consistent

Table 3-8
Third Party Reimbursement Elasticities

Occupation	Table and Regression Number	REIM Coefficient	Elasticity
Professional nurses	3-2(3)	5.28	0.03
	3-4(3)	7.92	0.04
Licensed practical nurses	3-2(6)	30.74	0.20
	3-4(7)	13.88	0.09
Medical technologists	3-2(9)	32.54	0.15
	3-4(11)	41.65	0.19
Transcribing machine operators	3-3(2)	9.56	0.06
	3-5(2)	21.16	0.14
Switchboard operators	3-2(4)	41.49	0.31
	3-5(5)	48.86	0.36
Aides-orderlies	3-3(6)	32.95	0.27
	3-5(8)	47.66	0.38
Porters-maids	3-3(8)	1.09	0.35
	3-5(11)	1.18	0.38

Table 3-9
Per-Capita Income Elasticities

Occupation	Table and Regression Number	INC Coefficient	Elasticity
Professional nurses	3-2(3)	0.017	0.42
	3-4(3)	0.023	0.56
Licensed practical nurses	3-2(6)	0.013	0.43
	3-4(7)	0.019	0.63
Medical technologists	3-2(9)	0.029	0.68
	3-4(11)	0.018	0.42
Transcribing machine operators	3-3(2)	0.014	0.47
	3-5(2)	0.022	0.75
Switchboard operators	3-3(4)	0.012	0.44
	3-5(5)	0.014	0.52
Aides-orderlies	3-3(6)	0.011	0.45
	3-5(8)	0.019	0.78
Porters-maids	3-3(8)	0.0003	0.49
	3-5(11)	0.0003	0.49

impacts on real hospital wages. The BEDS coefficients are often negative rather than positive, which would be the case if the variable were a "pure" demand variable. Negative signs on this type of variable have been interpreted in the past as evidence for the monopsony hypothesis (for example, Davis 1973). However, the variable is a crude proxy for the monopsony phenomenon at best. We prefer to infer from these regressions that BEDS has no systematic effect on hospital wages.

Conclusions and Implications

This chapter has examined the importance of several supply- and demand-side determinants   of real wages paid various types of hospital employees. It is evident that both kinds of factors have played a role in the increase in real hospital wages since 1960.

The estimated parameters and associated standard errors assist in identifying key behavioral relationships. They do not in and of themselves indicate which determinants played dominant roles at specific times within the 1960-1975 period. Since such demand side variables as real personal per capita income and the extent of third-party reimbursement grew at a much faster pace during the 1960s than during the first half of the 1970s, it is reasonable to infer that these types of factors were far more important driving forces behind the upward push in hospital wages during the earlier two-thirds of our observational period than subsequently. By contrast, the growth of hospital unions, a cost-push wage determinant, has been more pronounced during the 1970s. Thus, although developments on both sides of markets for hospital labor explain wage patterns, it is essential to recognize that the relative importance of specific factors has varied over time.

For all seven occupations evaluated, the variable representing the fraction of hospital employees covered by unions in the SMSA has a positive impact on wages. In the vast majority of cases, the estimated coefficient associated with the union variable is statistically significant (at the 5 percent level or higher). The coefficients suggest that a change from zero hospital union coverage in an SMSA to universal (100 percent) coverage raises wages from 4 to 18 percent on average. Transcribing machine and switchboard operators are at the low end; RNs are in the 6 to 7 percent range; LPNs, medical technologists, and aides-orderlies are at the high end. Politically, it may be impossible or undesirable for legislators to curb the growth of hospital unions. Yet when hospitals complain of cost pressures resulting from unionization, they do so with some justification.

Since the 1950s, there has been a growth in state minimum wage laws. From 1967 to the present, essentially all hospital workers have been covered under the federal minimum wage. According to conventional wisdom, every increase in the minimum wage is particularly burdensome on industries such as hospitals that are labor intensive and employ a high proportion of lower skilled persons. Furthermore, minimum wage increases affect higher- as well as lower-skilled employees because employers appear to try to maintain a relative wage structure. Minimum wage coefficients are consistently positive and statistically significant in the vast majority of regressions. Associated elasticities range from 0.05 to 0.15. This chapter's analysis implies that minimum wage increases boost hospital wages, although the effect is not dramatic. Again, it is unlikely that legislators can roll back minimum wages. Yet, when they raise the minimum, they should be aware that this has a positive effect on wages of both low- *and* high-skilled employees. Furthermore, by their actions, they are raising hospital costs.

High area unemployment rates may, in principle, temper hospital wage inflation, especially in the low-wage occupations. Our BLS analysis, however, reveals no effect. Poor results on this variable may be attributable to errors in variables in our unemployment rate series.

All forms of regulation, including occupational licensure, have come under increasing public scrutiny. Registered nurses and licensed practical nurses have been licensed for years. But there is a distinction between mandatory and permissive licensure: under the latter, only the title *RN* or *LPN* is protected; mandatory laws also define the scope of practice. The degree of specificity of such laws varies among states. Professional associations lobby for mandatory licensure on grounds of quality, but licensure also potentially offers financial advantages to the holders of the license. Our results suggest that mandatory licensure increases LPN wages by 5 to 6 percent. Medical technologists are licensed in a few states; we find a positive differential ranging up to 13 percent for licensed professionals in this occupation. We cannot judge the extent to which licensure has protected the public from incompetent providers, but some wage effects are indeed evident.

According to the traditional neoclassical models of the labor market, wage differentials for persons in a given skill-ability class in equilibrium are attributable to amenities of particular jobs and geographic locations. Holding occupation and industry constant, locational factors may be expected to be a much more important source of equilibrium wage differentials than job-specific amenities. Unfortunately, the list of potential amenity variables is almost endless. Certainly, there is no theory, in economics or in any other field, to serve as a guide. Both auto theft and homicide rates generally show positive impacts on wages, but the coefficients are generally insignificant at conventional levels. Economic theory provides no guide as to which amenity variables to include. It is impossible to rule out the possibility that important variables of this sort have been missed.

Past studies of wage determination in the hospital field have emphasized the role of monopsony power. Although some studies have assessed the monopsony issue in the context of wage setting of nonprofessional employees, there is widespread agreement that the monopsony concept is more applicable to professional employees. For purposes of this study we constructed three indexes of hospital bed and full-time equivalent employee concentration for the SMSAs in the BLS sample, using individual hospital records from AHA surveys. After constructing these indexes, it became readily apparent that all three are closely associated with city size. We cannot rule out the notion of monopsony power in hospital labor markets, but measures used to date do not show it very convincingly.

Most economists in recent years have tended to emphasize the role of demand-related factors as sources of hospital cost inflation in general and hospital wage inflation in particular. At the same time, developments on the factor supply side have been minimized. Our work suggests a definite role for some supply variables, especially unions. Minimum wages and licensure also contribute to increasing hospital wages.

We have also examined sources of wage inflation on the demand side. The enactment of Medicare and Medicaid in the mid-1960s meant a marked increase in the fraction of health care expenditures covered by third-party payors. We developed a time series of cross sections of average state, hospital-specific coinsurance rates for the years included in our analysis. Construction of these coinsurance rates involved several data sources and a number of assumptions. We have applied the estimated state rates to the SMSAs covered in the BLS sample. The estimated coefficients on the coinsurance rate variable are often statistically significant at conventional levels. As the fraction of hospital expense covered by private and governmental third parties rises, hospital wages rise. Associated elasticities range from 0.03 and 0.04 for RN wages to 0.38 for aides-orderlies and porters-maids. In general, elasticities for the lower skill categories are higher.

Rising hospital costs have also been attributed to increases in personal per capita income, and our research lends strong support to this view. Our real personal income measure consistently shows an effect on wages. Associated elasticities vary from 0.4 to 0.8.

Finally, studies of demand for hospital care generally include physician-population and bed-population ratios. In this chapter, these variables generally prove to be unimportant determinants of hospital wages.

Notes

1. See U.S. Bureau of Labor Statistics and U.S. Department of Health, Education, and Welfare (1968) and Kelly (1974).

2. See, for example, Davis (1973), Fein and Bishop (1976), Feldstein (1971), and Feldstein and Taylor (1977).

3. Feldstein (1971), Feldstein and Taylor (1977), Fottler (1977), Hurd (1973), and Salkever (1975).

4. Additional detail on the *Industry Wage Surveys* may be found in U.S. Department of Labor (1977).

5. See U.S. Department of Health, Education, and Welfare (1974) and our discussion of licensure that follows.

6. See, for example, Yett (1970).

7. Many, however, are members of unions.

8. The area price index is described in appendix A.

9. With the exception of the area price deflator, described in appendix A, additional information on construction of chapter 3 variables is found in appendix B.

10. See *Annual Digests of State and Federal Labor Legislation* published by the U.S. Bureau of Labor Standards.

11. Wage data are available for fewer than twenty-two SMSAs in 1960, but we have assembled (nonwage) data on all twenty-two SMSAs, irrespective of whether BLS wages are available for a given year.

12. In addition to the minimum wage studies cited, se also Kosters and Welch (1972), Mincer (1976), and, on employment effects, Welch (1977).

13. For example, see Livernash (1957).

14. Though perhaps tentative, their results are certainly interesting as a first approximation.

15. The possibility that unionization itself is endogenous has been explored more formally and extensively by Schmidt and Strauss (1976), Lee (1978), and Olsen (1978).

16. Her significant results notwithstanding, Sloan and Elnicki (1978) consulted individual state statutes and were unable to replicate Davis' labor law variable.

17. In two cases, it was difficult to determine from the state statute whether licensure for RNs was mandatory or permissive. We treated these as missing values in our regression analysis (for example, we excluded the cases entirely when a licensure variable was included). Here, these uncertain cases are part of the ten nonmandatory cases.

18. The same procedures outlined in note 17 have been followed.

19. Subcommittee on Health (1976).

20. See, for example, U.S. Environmental Protection Agency (1975).

21. Baird (1969).

22. See, for example, Feldstein (1971), and Salkever (1972).

23. We might have distinguished between specialist and generalist physicians and, in fact, do so in a later chapter. With our limited number of observations, we did not think the distinction was worth making in this chapter.

24. See Roemer (1961), and Roemer and Shain (1959).

25. See, for example, Rosenthal (1964), Feldstein (1971), Wennberg and Gittleson (1973), and McClure (1976).

26. Since AWAGE is in hourly terms in the aides-orderlies regressions and the dependent variable is expressed as a weekly wage, the parameter estimates sometimes are far in excess of 1. But if we divide AWAGE's parameters by forty to account for the difference in units, the resulting coefficients are far less than 1.

4

Are Hospitals Philanthropic Wage Setters? Evidence from the 1960 and 1970 U.S. Censuses

Introduction

The rapid rise in hospital wages during the 1960s has been well documented in chapter 3 and elsewhere.[1] By the late 1960s and early 1970s, hospital workers in some occupations and in some cities earned more than their counterparts in other industries.[2] Noting the rapid growth in hospital wages during the 1960s, Martin Feldstein (1971) developed the notion that hospitals are philanthropic wage setters as *one* explanation of this trend. In this chapter we question whether his hypothesis provides a good explanation of wage-setting patterns in the 1960s. Given the declines in real hospital wages during much of the 1970s, documented in chapters 1 and 3 and later in this book, it is very doubtful that one would construct such an hypothesis with hospital wage data now available. However, the issues Feldstein has raised are interesting ones and merit analysis beyond a mere look at trends.

According to Feldstein:

> The simplest economic logic requires that a profit-seeking firm should try to hire whatever group of workers it wants at lowest possible cost, i.e., it should never pay wage rates that are greater than levels necessary to hire these workers. The same principle is not at all compelling to the management of a nonprofit institution. A hospital, as a philanthropic or public organization, may concern itself with the welfare of its staff as well as of its patients. The tradition of low pay for hospital staff developed when hospital budgets were very tight and the institutions were largely dependent on voluntary philanthropic support. More recently, the rapid rise in the demand for hospital care has given hospital administrators much greater freedom in determining salary levels .... A ... way in which hospitals could and, I believe, have used their increased discretionary financial power has been by raising the wages of hospital personnel above the levels necessary to obtain the staff they wanted. ... Although hospital administrators might dislike the notion that they have willingly contributed to unnecessary increases in hospital costs, they would defend the practice of paying "decent" and "just" wages rather than the lowest wages at which the services could be obtained (p. 68).

Whether the philanthropic motive provides an important explanation of hospital wage inflation at any time in our recent history is far more than a

49

scholarly issue. There is undoubtedly widespread agreement that the primary reason for increased government financing in the health care field is to improve access to health care services. To the extent that the public desires to transfer income from one group of citizens to another, few would want to charge health service providers or any other employer with this responsibility. If hospitals are paying wage rates above the level necessary to attract employees, this is information many third-party payors, especially those paying "reasonable" costs, would certainly like to have.

There are several reasons, other than a philanthropic motive, that might lead an employer to pay more than the lowest wage in a given occupation. As noted in chapter 2, higher wages may reduce turnover and hence specific training costs employers incur (Pencavel 1970, 1972; Parsons 1972; Nickell 1976). However, previous studies on turnover rates of professional nurses in hospitals by Elnicki and Sloan (1975) and Sloan (1978) indicate that nurse turnover is quite unresponsive to changes in wages. Thus this matter is not pursued further here.[3] Higher pay may increase job satisfaction and thereby boost productivity. There has been some research on job satisfaction in nursing (among hospital occupations), but this topic, too, is beyond the scope of our study.[4] To attract workers above the minimum quality level in a given occupation, it is necessary to pay higher wages. If aspects of the job are particularly undesirable and/or risky, a "compensating" wage differential may be required (Thaler and Rosen 1975). Firms desiring to expand their work forces at an unusually rapid pace may have to pay higher than normal wages to overcome transactions costs workers incur by changing jobs. However, the compensating wage differentials argument cannot explain the *growth* in wages; nor do available data permit us to link wage change to transactions costs. On the other hand, the census data are especially appropriate for assessing the impact of third-party reimbursement on the quality of the hospital work force. This potential relationship is evaluated here as an alternative to the philanthropic explanation of wage trends observed during the 1960s.

This chapter's empirical work consists of two parts. First, using microdata from the 1 percent samples of the 1960 and 1970 U.S. censuses of population, we compare wage rates in hospitals with three reference-group industries. A rather straightforward method allows us to partition wage differentials into two component parts: a quality difference between the hospital work force and each of the reference groups; and a quality-adjusted wage difference. If hospitals are indeed philanthropists, they should pay more than other industries holding quality constant—the quality-adjusted wage difference.

The second part, based exclusively on hospital data with states as observational units from the same census sources, investigates the following seven hypotheses:

1. Work-force quality is a normal good—that is, higher quality will be demanded in states with more generous third-party reimbursement for hospital services and higher levels of personal per capita income.

2. The "own" quality-adjusted wage effect on quality is negative—that is, in states which pay higher quality-adjusted wages, we hypothesize that hospitals, other things being equal, purchase less quality (a downward-sloping demand curve for quality).
3. Quality-adjusted wages are higher in states with substantial amounts of hospital union activity, as measured by the fraction of hospitals with a union contract, with strike activity, and which have had requests for recognition by a union (within the past year).
4. Minimum wages raise quality-adjusted wages (only tested for 1960).
5. Quality-adjusted wages partly reflect the tightness of state labor markets as measured by the state unemployment rate.
6. Labor markets take a long time to clear. Hence, in state cross-sectional analysis of quality-adjusted wages, there is a role for variables influencing the demand for the hospital's product. In chapter 3, a definite role was found for demand variables as wage determinants. We have made, however, a more concerted effort to hold worker quality characteristics constant in this chapter.
7. Quality-adjusted wages are highest in states in which the 1965-1970 growth of hospital work force was the most rapid.

When we discuss work-force "quality" throughout this chapter, we refer to employee characteristics that are highly valued by the market. The market's values may in some cases reflect prejudice; some types of workers may systematically receive lower wages because of discrimination. By no means do we endorse discrimination; we report what the market *does* value, not what it *should* value.

Comparisons between Hospital and Reference Industries Wages

Selecting Reference Groups

In previous studies by Feldstein (1971) and Fuchs (1976), hospital employees' wages have been compared to those of nonagricultural workers outside the health field. Research by proponents of the segmented labor markets theory and others has demonstrated rather convincingly that interindustry wage differentials persist, even after one controls for numerous characteristics of workers in each of the industries.[5] Given persistent interindustry differences, one is likely to learn more by comparing hospital wages with wages in reasonably homogeneous clusters of industries than with means for the nonagricultural work force as a whole.

Using notions developed by such nonneoclassical labor economists as Clark Kerr, Peter Doeringer, and Michael Piore,[6] Arthur Alexander (1974) classified industries as "manorial," "guild," or "unstructured." In a manorial firm, there is a substantial amount of firm-specific training; promotion ladders are well-defined and reflect the gradual accumulation of firm-specific human capital. With a well-defined labor market internal to the firm, a characteristic of manorial industries, there is a relatively low probability of an employee leaving the organization.

Guild industries typically employ workers with substantial skills in the crafts. Human capital is industry specific rather than firm specific; as a result, worker loyalty is to the craft or industry rather than to the firm. In guild industries, there is substantial interfirm, but comparatively little interindustry mobility.

Unstructured industries offer employees limited opportunities for either general or firm-specific skill acquisition. As a result, ties to both firms and industries are relatively weak, and interfirm *and* interindustry mobility are correspondingly high. In segmented labor market terminology, one could safely characterize manorial as operating in primary labor markets, and unstructured firms as operating in secondary labor markets.

Alexander developed an empirical method for classifying four-digit Standard Industrial Classification (SIC) industries into one of the three categories, based on interindustry and interfirm mobility patterns observed in the social security 1 percent work history file for the years 1957-1966. During this period, the file contained job tenure information on approximately one million individuals. An in-depth discussion of Alexander's methods would take us too far afield, but it is useful to consider examples of industries falling into each of Alexander's three classes:

Manorial	missiles and space vehicles; petroleum refining; tires and tubes; aircraft engines; motor vehicles; telephone communications; gas companies; "combined" utilities.
Guild	highway construction; plumbing, heating, and air-conditioning contractors; painting and papering contractors; barber shops; scrap and waste wholesale; motor vehicle dealers.
Unstructured	millwork plants; footwear; department stores; grocery stores; drug stores; wood household furniture; hospitals.

Judging from Alexander's results, during the years 1957-1966 hospitals exhibited features of firms in unstructured industries. However, increased third-party reimbursement, especially since 1966, the year in which Medicare and Medicaid took effect, may have changed their classification.

Unfortunately, the census uses a three- rather than a four-digit code; for this reason, we were not able to find matches for each of the industries classified by Alexander as being either manorial, guild, or unstructured. Furthermore, since there are some differences in the census industry codes for 1960 and 1970, the names of industries presented in appendix E differ somewhat from Alexander's, but we believe not in important ways.

Method of Decomposing Hospital-Nonhospital
Wage Differences into Work-Force Quality
and Quality-Adjusted Wage Components

Hospital-reference industry wage differences may be divided into a component attributable to work-force quality, and a quality-adjusted wage component, according to:

$$\frac{w_{ht}\,(\bar{h})}{w_{rt}\,(\bar{r})} = \frac{w_{ht}\,(\bar{h})}{w_{rt}\,(\bar{h})} \bullet \frac{w_{rt}\,(\bar{h})}{w_{rt}\,(\bar{r})} \quad \text{or} \tag{4.1}$$

| crude wage difference | quality-adjusted wage difference | quality difference |

$$\frac{w_{ht}\,(\bar{h})}{w_{rt}\,(\bar{r})} = \frac{w_{ht}\,(\bar{h})}{w_{ht}\,(\bar{r})} \bullet \frac{w_{ht}\,(\bar{r})}{w_{rt}\,(\bar{r})} \tag{4.2}$$

| crude wage difference | quality difference | quality-adjusted wage difference |

where

w = hourly wage rate or annual earnings

$\bar{h}$ = characteristics of hospital workers (mean values)

$\bar{r}$ = characteristics of reference group workers [either manorial (m), guild (g), or unstructured (u) mean values]

t = 1960 or 1970

Equation 4.1 states that the ratio of the observed hospital wage rate to the observed reference industry wage rate is the product of the ratio of the observed hospital wage and the wage that hospital workers would receive if they were paid on the same basis as reference industry workers, and the ratio of the wage that hospital workers would receive if they were paid on the same basis as reference workers and the observed reference industry wage. The first ratio on the right side of equation 4.1 is a "pure" or quality-adjusted wage differential; both numerator and denominator pertain to a work force (hospital) with a common set of characteristics. The second ratio reflects worker quality, since it uses a common wage-setting structure (for the reference industry) and work forces with varying characteristics (hospital and reference).

Equation 4.2 bases the quality-adjusted wage difference on characteristics of the reference industry work force. Although both equations 4.1 and 4.2 are correct algebraically, empirical estimates of pure wage and quality components vary slightly depending on which formula is used; we present results based on both.

Previous research by Feldstein (1971) and Fuchs (1976) attempted to hold worker characteristics constant by stratifying by occupation (Feldstein), or by color, sex, age, and schooling (Fuchs). Fein and Bishop (1976) have presented interesting descriptive evidence on hospital work-force composition in tabular form. However, a far more precise decomposition of pure wage and quality differences can be obtained with regression analysis. To ascertain differences in wage-setting structure in 1960 and 1970 in hospitals and the three reference industries by sex, we have specified and estimated sixteen hourly wage regressions.[7]

Hourly Wage Equation Specification

Economists now have considerable experience in specifying and estimating wage-generating equations. For this reason, our discussion is limited to a few salient features of our specification and empirical results. Brief definitions of explanatory variables are presented in table 4-1. Since the 1970 census contains several pertinent explanatory variables unavailable for 1960, the specification for the two years, although similar, is not identical.

Using the theory of investment in human capital, Mincer (1970, 1974) demonstrated that wage equations in a semi-log form (natural log for the wage and a linear form for the explanatory variables) have some desirable theoretical features under certain conditions. Mincer's functional form is employed here. Wages have been deflated by an area price index;[8] both 1960 and 1970 wages are in 1960 dollars.

The 1960 and 1970 equations contain variables for schooling (EDUC and EDUCSQ), employment experience (EXPER and EXPSQ, NMARR and UMARR,[9] and CLT2 through CLT19), race-ethnicity (FR1, FR2, BLACK, SPANAME, and BC[10]), and location (RESMT, URB, previous residence—RES55 or RES65, and census division NE through MT, with Pacific the omitted category).

Table 4-1
Definitions of Explanatory Variables

Variable Name	Definition
BC	Equals one if black *and* born in a state of the old Confederacy
BLACK	Equals one if black
CLT2	Number of children in household under age two
CLT6	Number of children in household ages two to five
CLT16	Number of children in household ages six to fifteen
CLT19	Number of children in household ages sixteen to eighteen
DISLIM1	Equals one if disability limits work but does not prevent work *and* has lasted two years or less
DISLIM2	Same as DISLIM1 except disability has been of more than two years duration
EARN	Individual's annual earnings in 1959 (1969) divided by area price index
EDUC (EDSQ)	Years of schooling (years squared)
ENC	East North Central census division
ESC	East South Central census division
EXPER (EXPSQ)	Years of experience in work force (experience years squared)
FR1	Equals one if foreign born, but from English-speaking or Western European country
FR2	Equals one if foreign born, and not from countries included in FR1
FR3	Equals one if foreign born (either FR1 or FR2), but immigrated to United States in 1968 or earlier
GULD	Person works in a "guild" industry
HW	Individual's hourly wage–constructed as annual earnings in 1959 (1969) divided by product of (a) weeks worked in 1959 (1969), (b) hours worked during 1960 (1970) reference week and (c) area price index
HOSP	Person works in hospital
IND65	Equals one if person's 1965 industry differs from his 1970 industry and WORK65 = 1
MA	Mid-Atlantic census division
MNOR	Person works in a "manorial" industry
MT	Mountain census division
NE	Northeast census division
NMARR	Equals one if never married
NVOC	Equals one if person has received *no* vocational training
OCC65	Equals one if person's 1965 occupation differs from his 1970 occupation and WORK65 = 1
RESMT	Equals one for resident of metropolitan areas
RES55(65)	Equals one if person's 1960 (1970) state of residence differs from state of residence in 1955 (1965)
SA	South Atlantic census division
SPANAME	Equals one if Spanish surname
UMARR	Equals one if widowed, separated, or divorced in 1960 (1970)
UNST	Person works in an unstructured industry
URB	Equals one if resident of urban, nonmetropolitan areas
WKCC	Equals one if person works in central city of metropolitan area
WNC	West North Central census division
WORK65	Equals one if person worked at job or business in 1965
WSC	West South Central census division

The 1960 specification contains one unique variable, WKCC, which equals one if the individual works in a central city of a metropolitan area. Several variables are only available for 1970. To measure vocational training, NVOC equals one if the individual has had no such training. There are two variables for disability (DISLIM1 and DISLIM2) and three additional measures of work experience (WORK 65 = 1 if person was employed in 1965, OCC65 if 1965 and 1970 occupations are not the same and WORK65 = 1, and IND65 if 1965 and 1970 industries are not the same and WORK65 = 1). A binary variable FR3 identifies foreign-born persons who immigrated to the United States more than two years before the census.

In both years, we selected employed persons aged eighteen to sixty-four, living in the coterminous United States, with five years of college or less, and with hourly wages between $0.65 and $25.00 (in 1960 dollars). All self-employed persons and persons with doctorates (and a high proportion of those with masters degrees) have been excluded.

Means of Variables and Estimated
Hourly Wage Regressions

Tables 4-2 and 4-3 present means of explanatory variables for 1960 and 1970, respectively. A few aspects of the means are particularly noteworthy. For both years and sexes, employees in manorial industries had both the highest hourly wages and annual earnings. In 1960, male hospital workers had by far the lowest real hourly wages (see HW) and real annual earnings (see EARN) of the four industry groups; although below manorial workers, female hospital employees had higher wages and earnings than their counterparts in either guild or unstructured industries. By 1970, male hospital workers had surpassed their peers in unstructured industries in terms of annual earnings, but not in terms of the hourly wage. The relative position of female hospital employees was the same in 1970 as in 1960.

Summary measures of worker characteristics will be presented later. However, some interesting patterns in specific characteristics are revealed in tables 4-2 and 4-3. Female hospital workers had higher mean years of schooling (EDUC) than either females or males in the three other industries in both 1960 and 1970. Male hospital employees had less schooling on the average than males in either manorial or unstructured industries in 1960; but by 1970, they were virtually tied with male manorial employees and slightly above male and female workers in the other two industry categories. In 1970, both male and female hospital employees led the others in the proportions of the work force with some type of vocation training (NVOC = 1 if persons received no vocational training).

Judging from all means of the variable BLACK, the fraction of black employees was substantially higher in hospitals than in the other industry

Table 4-2
Means of Explanatory Variables, 1960

Variable	Males				Females			
	HOSP	MNOR	GULD	UNST	HOSP	MNOR	GULD	UNST
WKCC	0.51	0.43	0.49	0.46	0.53	0.54	0.62	0.57
RESMT	0.70	0.77	0.68	0.64	0.67	0.77	0.75	0.72
URB	0.16	0.13	0.17	0.20	0.21	0.15	0.17	0.18
BLACK	0.21	0.07	0.10	0.08	0.12	0.03	0.10	0.04
SPANAME	0.06	0.04	0.08	0.05	0.10	0.07	0.10	0.07
EXPER	27.5	26.7	26.5	26.2	25.5	21.5	27.0	28.4
NMARR	0.19	0.09	0.13	0.11	0.23	0.23	0.16	0.13
UMARR	0.15	0.08	0.11	0.09	0.32	0.21	0.36	0.31
FR1	0.07	0.05	0.05	0.04	0.06	0.04	0.05	0.05
FR2	0.05	0.04	0.06	0.05	0.03	0.02	0.04	0.03
BC	0.13	0.05	0.08	0.06	0.08	0.02	0.07	0.02
EDUC	9.95	10.45	9.91	10.22	11.69	11.34	10.43	10.60
RES55	0.09	0.07	0.09	0.07	0.10	0.08	0.08	0.05
CLT2	0.04	0.03	0.04	0.03	0.01	0.0045	0.01	0.0031
CLT6	0.06	0.08	0.08	0.08	0.03	0.02	0.03	0.01
CLT16	0.16	0.21	0.22	0.23	0.11	0.07	0.12	0.09
CLT19	0.08	0.12	0.11	0.14	0.07	0.07	0.09	0.09
NE	0.08	0.06	0.06	0.08	0.07	0.07	0.05	0.08
MA	0.34	0.23	0.26	0.24	0.26	0.28	0.27	0.24
ENC	0.18	0.34	0.17	0.18	0.20	0.25	0.21	0.21
WNC	0.07	0.05	0.07	0.08	0.10	0.07	0.09	0.10
SA	0.09	0.06	0.10	0.10	0.08	0.07	0.08	0.09
ESC	0.04	0.03	0.05	0.06	0.04	0.03	0.03	0.05
WSC	0.07	0.07	0.10	0.09	0.06	0.06	0.08	0.07
MT	0.03	0.02	0.05	0.03	0.04	0.03	0.05	0.03
HW	1.89	3.02	2.57	2.37	1.70	2.12	1.60	1.62
EARN	3864.9	6004.5	4917.7	5095.7	3081.10	3994.2	2782.7	2852.2
Number of observations	762	11,492	10,178	5,773	2,799	3,527	4,756	3,810

groupings. This finding cannot be explained by differences in community size or in the distribution of employees by Census Division.

The experience measure (EXPER) reflects age and years of schooling completed. Younger workers tend to have had more formal schooling than older workers. At the same time, years in schooling represent a deduction from years in the work force. As defined, this variable is far more descriptive of male than female work experience, since males tend to work more continuously than females, and EXPER assumes (necessarily) continuous employment.[11] There are no meaningful interindustry differences in EXPER. The 1970 census requested information on work activity (WORK65), industry (IND65), and occupation (OCC65) in 1965. Judging by the means of these variables, hospital and manorial workers had somewhat less work-, industry-, and occupation-specific experience on the average than did guild and unstructured workers. These differences may

Table 4-3
Means of Explanatory Variables, 1970

Variable	Males				Females			
	HOSP	*MNOR*	*GULD*	*UNST*	*HOSP*	*MNOR*	*GULD*	*UNST*
RESMT	0.68	0.75	0.64	0.64	0.68	0.78	0.70	0.63
URB	0.19	0.14	0.17	0.19	0.18	0.14	0.17	0.20
BLACK	0.18	0.10	0.10	0.08	0.17	0.09	0.10	0.04
SPANAME	0.04	0.02	0.03	0.04	0.03	0.02	0.03	0.03
EXPER	20.73	19.65	18.28	15.84	19.85	16.23	20.02	19.43
NMARR	0.26	0.21	0.32	0.42	0.23	0.35	0.23	0.27
UMARR	0.11	0.12	0.12	0.11	0.26	0.17	0.22	0.19
FR1	0.01	0.02	0.02	0.02	0.03	0.03	0.03	0.02
FR2	0.03	0.02	0.03	0.02	0.02	0.01	0.02	0.01
BC	0.11	0.06	0.07	0.05	0.12	0.04	0.07	0.03
EDUC	11.82	11.83	11.22	11.54	12.18	11.95	11.30	11.46
WORK65	0.88	0.88	0.93	0.92	0.91	0.94	0.97	0.96
FR3	0.03	0.04	0.03	0.03	0.04	0.03	0.04	0.03
NVOC	0.62	0.66	0.72	0.76	0.48	0.75	0.79	0.79
DISLIM1	0.04	0.02	0.02	0.01	0.02	0.01	0.02	0.02
DISLIM2	0.06	0.06	0.06	0.06	0.03	0.01	0.03	0.02
RES65	0.08	0.07	0.07	0.06	0.09	0.06	0.08	0.06
IND65	0.39	0.34	0.46	0.49	0.47	0.51	0.58	0.58
OCC65	0.40	0.43	0.52	0.59	0.49	0.57	0.63	0.67
CLT2	0.09	0.12	0.09	0.08	0.05	0.03	0.05	0.03
CLT6	0.17	0.19	0.18	0.15	0.14	0.12	0.14	0.12
CLT16	0.52	0.51	0.55	0.65	0.63	0.53	0.62	0.67
CLT19	0.18	0.19	0.23	0.32	0.23	0.22	0.24	0.26
NE	0.10	0.06	0.06	0.07	0.08	0.06	0.06	0.09
MA	0.21	0.18	0.18	0.17	0.20	0.17	0.17	0.17
ENC	0.18	0.34	0.17	0.18	0.18	0.31	0.23	0.22
WNC	0.08	0.05	0.07	0.09	0.10	0.06	0.08	0.09
SA	0.11	0.10	0.18	0.17	0.13	0.11	0.15	0.12
ESC	0.07	0.06	0.06	0.07	0.05	0.04	0.05	0.07
WSC	0.10	0.07	0.10	0.09	0.09	0.09	0.10	0.10
MT	0.02	0.03	0.04	0.04	0.04	0.02	0.04	0.04
HW	2.49	3.46	2.85	2.56	2.20	2.41	1.91	1.91
EARN	4917	6809	5464	4890	3661	4204	2882	3032
Number of observations	340	1,627	2,749	1,548	1,314	895	1,673	910

reflect differential rates of growth in industry work forces rather than characteristics intrinsic to the industries themselves.

Tables 4-4 and 4-5 present estimated hourly wage-generating functions for 1960 and 1970, respectively. The R^2s range from 0.09 to 0.37. Although most of the variance in the wages remains unexplained, R^2s in this range are common with microdata. R^2s associated with annual earnings regressions presented in appendix F tend to be substantially higher than those in tables 4-4 and 4-5. Since the earnings regressions contain the same explanatory variables as their wage counterparts, it is reasonable to attribute the lower R^2s in tables 4-4 and 4-5, at least in part, to errors in the wage dependent variables. As described in table 4-1, the wage variable (HW) is based on earnings in the previous year divided by the product of weeks worked in the previous year and hours worked during a reference week in the census year. Specifically, work hours in the reference week may in some cases have been atypical and unrepresentative of work activity in the previous year.

Tests for regression coefficient homogeneity reveal statistically significant differences in wage-generating structure in all cases; however, it is usual to find statistical significance when regressions are based on very large samples. Significance levels on individual coefficients are not presented to avoid clutter in the tables.

These are the principal findings from the wage regression analysis. The estimated wage functions allow one to calculate rates of return to schooling, using the EDUC and EDUCSQ coefficients. Evaluated at twelve years of schooling, the payoff in terms of increased wages is slightly higher in hospitals than in the reference industries. Even for hospital workers, the returns are low, 3.3 and 1.7 percent at the margin for males in 1960 and 1979, and 1.7 and 1.5 percent for females in these years. Estimated marginal rates of return rise monotonically with years of schooling completed. For example, at sixteen years, the 1970 rate is 3.1 percent, versus 1.7 percent at twelve years.

Judging from the NVOC coefficients, the payoff from a vocational program tends to be higher than returns from a comparable amount of formal education. Assume, for example, in the case of female hospital workers, that the vocational program is a diploma nursing program lasting three years. Then, taking the NVOC parameter in table 4-5 of −0.113 and dividing by three, the annualized rate of return in the hospital sector is 3.8 for the high-school graduate in 1970 versus 1.5 percent from an additional year of formal schooling. Of course, a typical vocational program does not last three years. If anything, the 3.8 figure is an underestimate of the return to females in the hospital sector. As with formal education, the payoff to vocational training tends to be higher in the hospital sector than in the reference industries.

Unlike schooling, the marginal return to an additional year of work experience declines with the number of years of experience. Estimated returns are remarkably stable between 1960 and 1970, but tend to be higher for males than for females. The higher estimated marginal payoff for males is not too surprising because, as previously noted, the experience variable is a far better measure for males than females. Interindustry differences in the marginal returns to work experience, gauged by the EXPER and EXPSQ coefficient, are negligible.

Work experience is also captured in 1970 by dummy variables WORK65, IND65, and OCC65. That an individual worked in another industry in 1965 (IND65 = 1) has important effects on wages in hospital, manorial, and guild regressions for males; for females, the coefficient of WORK65 is statistically significant (and large) only in the manorial industry regression.

Judging from the industry variables, industry-specific experience has

Table 4-4
Wage Regressions, 1960

Variable	Males				Females			
	HOSP	MNOR	GULD	UNST	HOSP	MNOR	GULD	UNST
WKCC	-0.040 (0.033)	-0.017 (0.0073)	-0.027 (0.011)	0.013 (0.013)	0.027 (0.017)	0.0064 (0.013)	0.040 (0.015)	0.046 (0.015)
RESMT	0.064 (0.046)	0.088 (0.012)	0.152 (0.016)	0.151 (0.019)	0.047 (0.025)	0.110 (0.023)	0.091 (0.025)	0.052 (0.023)
URB	0.041 (0.048)	0.056 (0.014)	0.052 (0.017)	0.086 (0.018)	0.038 (0.025)	0.060 (0.025)	0.023 (0.025)	0.014 (0.023)
BLACK	-0.158 (0.051)	-0.180 (0.026)	-0.225 (0.030)	-0.172 (0.042)	-0.073 (0.032)	-0.069 (0.051)	-0.152 (0.034)	-0.106 (0.043)
SPANAME	-0.086 (0.063)	0.0080 (0.018)	-0.126 (0.020)	-0.045 (0.028)	0.064 (0.029)	0.032 (0.027)	0.060 (0.024)	-0.00051 (0.027)
EXPER	0.024 (0.0039)	0.029 (0.0011)	0.025 (0.0014)	0.029 (0.0016)	0.0093 (0.0020)	0.019 (0.0016)	0.0067 (0.0018)	0.0097 (0.0019)
EXPSQ	-0.00038 (0.00007)	-0.00039 (0.00002)	-0.00040 (0.00003)	-0.00045 (0.00003)	-0.00015 (0.00004)	-0.00031 (0.00003)	-0.00012 (0.00004)	-0.00022 (0.00004)
NMARR	-0.027 (0.038)	-0.080 (0.012)	-0.133 (0.016)	-0.082 (0.019)	0.018 (0.019)	0.061 (0.015)	0.071 (0.018)	0.101 (0.019)
UMARR	-0.082 (0.039)	-0.053 (0.012)	-0.070 (0.016)	-0.074 (0.019)	-0.033 (0.017)	0.022 (0.015)	-0.00030 (0.014)	0.0011 (0.014)
FR1	0.030 (0.054)	-0.010 (0.016)	-0.012 (0.023)	0.052 (0.028)	-0.030 (0.028)	-0.030 (0.029)	-0.027 (0.026)	-0.035 (0.026)
FR2	-0.058 (0.064)	-0.018 (0.017)	-0.108 (0.021)	-0.030 (0.027)	-0.093 (0.044)	-0.094 (0.042)	-0.024 (0.030)	-0.0043 (0.035)
BC	0.110 (0.061)	0.0083 (0.030)	-0.051 (0.034)	-0.096 (0.047)	-0.054 (0.039)	-0.091 (0.067)	-0.036 (0.039)	-0.152 (0.059)
EDUC	0.011 (0.019)	-0.025 (0.0055)	-0.027 (0.0062)	-0.037 (0.0079)	-0.00097 (0.013)	-0.022 (0.013)	-0.029 (0.010)	-0.054 (0.013)
EDSQ	0.0014 (0.00088)	0.0032 (0.00026)	0.0031 (0.00031)	0.0037 (0.00039)	0.0023 (0.00058)	0.0024 (0.00062)	0.0035 (0.00052)	0.0034 (0.00064)

	(1)	(2)	(3)	(4)	(5)	(6)	(7)	(8)
RES55	-0.046 (0.047)	-0.0070 (0.013)	0.015 (0.017)	0.064 (0.022)	-0.00024 (0.023)	-0.014 (0.021)	-0.026 (0.022)	-0.043 (0.026)
CLT2	-0.114 (0.072)	0.017 (0.018)	-0.021 (0.023)	0.026 (0.029)	0.105 (0.057)	0.0026 (0.079)	0.017 (0.059)	-0.113 (0.100)
CLT6	0.092 (0.054)	0.010 (0.011)	0.00084 (0.015)	0.016 (0.017)	0.017 (0.035)	-0.041 (0.035)	-0.017 (0.033)	0.037 (0.038)
CLT16	-0.014 (0.022)	0.0073 (0.0052)	0.016 (0.0069)	0.0082 (0.0081)	0.048 (0.015)	-0.043 (0.015)	0.0057 (0.013)	-0.017 (0.015)
CLT19	0.071 (0.048)	0.0094 (0.0093)	0.061 (0.014)	0.0072 (0.014)	0.030 (0.024)	-0.065 (0.020)	-0.047 (0.019)	-0.021 (0.019)
NE	-0.150 (0.065)	-0.190 (0.016)	-0.210 (0.024)	-0.228 (0.024)	-0.108 (0.033)	-0.174 (0.028)	-0.189 (0.032)	-0.218 (0.028)
MA	-0.059 (0.049)	-0.040 (0.012)	-0.126 (0.016)	-0.130 (0.019)	-0.029 (0.026)	-0.030 (0.021)	-0.034 (0.022)	-0.124 (0.022)
ENC	0.125 (0.053)	0.049 (0.011)	-0.017 (0.018)	-0.040 (0.019)	-0.0018 (0.026)	0.031 (0.021)	-0.016 (0.022)	-0.077 (0.022)
WNC	-0.070 (0.066)	-0.029 (0.018)	-0.157 (0.022)	-0.184 (0.024)	-0.100 (0.030)	-0.055 (0.027)	-0.090 (0.027)	-0.159 (0.026)
SA	-0.066 (0.063)	0.075 (0.017)	-0.155 (0.020)	-0.138 (0.023)	-0.024 (0.032)	0.091 (0.027)	-0.047 (0.028)	-0.133 (0.027)
ESC	-0.177 (0.080)	0.021 (0.020)	-0.181 (0.026)	-0.180 (0.027)	-0.055 (0.040)	-0.014 (0.035)	-0.104 (0.037)	-0.125 (0.032)
WSC	-0.132 (0.065)	0.042 (0.016)	-0.176 (0.020)	-0.187 (0.023)	-0.158 (0.032)	-0.080 (0.027)	-0.088 (0.026)	-0.186 (0.027)
MT	0.053 (0.094)	0.033 (0.027)	-0.017 (0.027)	-0.051 (0.035)	-0.030 (0.041)	-0.0048 (0.041)	-0.047 (0.035)	-0.043 (0.041)
CONSTANT	0.021	0.435	0.497	0.361	0.026	0.296	0.148	0.553
	$R^2 = 0.24$ $F(27,734)$ $= 8.58$	$R^2 = 0.20$ $F(27,115)$ $= 104.46$	$R^2 = 0.15$ $F(27,102)$ $= 68.19$	$R^2 = 0.20$ $F(27,575)$ $= 53.69$	$R^2 = 0.18$ $F(27,277)$ $= 23.24$	$R^2 = 0.14$ $F(27,3499)$ $= 21.50$	$R^2 = 0.13$ $F(27,4728)$ $= 26.24$	$R^2 = 0.09$ $F(27,3782)$ $= 14.08$

Note: Figures in parentheses are standard errors.

Table 4-5
Wage Regressions, 1970

Variable	Males				Females			
	HOSP	MNOR	GULD	UNST	HOSP	MNOR	GULD	UNST
RESMT	0.115 (0.065)	0.019 (0.033)	0.024 (0.025)	0.089 (0.033)	0.083 (0.034)	0.036 (0.049)	0.012 (0.034)	0.085 (0.037)
URB	0.042 (0.074)	0.026 (0.040)	0.088 (0.030)	0.063 (0.039)	0.119 (0.040)	0.004: (0.057)	0.034 (0.040)	0.112 (0.043)
BLACK	-0.048 (0.083)	-0.257 (0.049)	-0.162 (0.054)	-0.098 (0.073)	-0.101 (0.052)	-0.117 (0.065)	-0.109 (0.060)	-0.066 (0.126)
SPANAME	-0.107 (0.114)	-0.121 (0.064)	-0.120 (0.053)	-0.003 (0.065)	-0.173 (0.075)	-0.055 (0.089)	-0.109 (0.064)	0.094 (0.086)
EXPER	0.023 (0.0060)	0.023 (0.0031)	0.023 (0.0030)	0.015 (0.0036)	0.016 (0.0035)	0.016 (0.0041)	0.011 (0.003)	0.011 (0.004)
EXPSQ	-0.00038 (0.00012)	-0.00034 (0.00007)	-0.00042 (0.00006)	-0.00021 (0.00008)	-0.00031 (0.00008)	-0.00026 (0.00010)	-0.00027 (0.00007)	-0.00023 (0.00009)
NMARR	-0.154 (0.060)	-0.085 (0.030)	-0.191 (0.028)	-0.193 (0.037)	0.057 (0.032)	0.071 (0.033)	0.0052 (0.034)	0.093 (0.039)
UMARR	-0.101 (0.060)	0.029 (0.030)	0.084 (0.028)	-0.057 (0.037)	-0.012 (0.032)	0.054 (0.033)	0.033 (0.034)	-0.034 (0.039)
FR1	-0.0075 (0.206)	0.060 (0.127)	-0.0077 (0.091)	0.123 (0.135)	0.218 (0.127)	0.117 (0.163)	-0.099 (0.149)	-0.120 (0.211)
FR2	0.034 (0.191)	-0.148 (0.115)	-0.054 (0.085)	0.098 (0.106)	0.090 (0.116)	0.149 (0.185)	0.036 (0.136)	-0.187 (0.065)
BC	-0.090 (0.101)	0.107 (0.063)	0.013 (0.063)	-0.079 (0.088)	-0.053 (0.059)	0.014 (0.088)	0.049 (0.072)	0.050 (0.149)
EDUC	-0.025 (0.034)	-0.039 (0.021)	-0.031 (0.016)	-0.050 (0.023)	-0.035 (0.023)	-0.065 (0.037)	-0.081 (0.026)	-0.142 (0.040)

	(1)	(2)	(3)	(4)	(5)	(6)	(7)	(8)
EDSQ	0.0080 (0.0019)	0.0056 (0.0013)	0.0043 (0.0017)	0.0042 (0.0010)	0.0039 (0.0010)	0.0040 (0.00076)	0.0040 (0.00092)	0.0035 (0.0014)
WORK65	0.029 (0.080)	0.076 (0.068)	0.184 (0.066)	-0.035 (0.046)	0.011 (0.051)	0.162 (0.041)	0.087 (0.038)	0.192 (0.080)
FR3	0.369 (0.202)	0.120 (0.146)	-0.068 (0.171)	-0.066 (0.125)	-0.118 (0.125)	0.064 (0.090)	0.066 (0.122)	0.192 (0.207)
NVOC	0.00011 (0.033)	-0.103 (0.027)	-0.040 (0.030)	-0.113 (0.023)	-0.042 (0.028)	-0.087 (0.021)	-0.013 (0.021)	-0.077 (0.044)
DISLIM1	0.169 (0.103)	-0.085 (0.081)	-0.036 (0.122)	-0.055 (0.081)	0.191 (0.095)	-0.088 (0.060)	-0.058 (0.063)	-0.150 (0.103)
DISLIM2	0.134 (0.093)	-0.067 (0.062)	0.038 (0.107)	0.031 (0.071)	-0.077 (0.048)	-0.087 (0.037)	-0.030 (0.041)	-0.037 (0.083)
RES65	-0.022 (0.057)	0.059 (0.042)	-0.025 (0.056)	-0.00021 (0.039)	0.026 (0.049)	0.043 (0.036)	0.073 (0.039)	0.022 (0.079)
IND65	-0.005 (0.038)	0.0063 (0.033)	-0.156 (0.038)	-0.066 (0.037)	-0.038 (0.034)	-0.075 (0.027)	-0.111 (0.029)	-0.025 (0.063)
OCC65	-0.165 (0.037)	-0.045 (0.032)	-0.029 (0.037)	-0.089 (0.037)	-0.090 (0.032)	-0.054 (0.026)	0.00036 (0.027)	-0.135 (0.063)
CLT2	0.079 (0.077)	0.083 (0.050)	-0.026 (0.069)	0.050 (0.052)	0.014 (0.045)	0.013 (0.031)	-0.00049 (0.030)	-0.102 (0.074)
CLT6	0.057 (0.035)	0.0032 (0.028)	0.084 (0.036)	-0.011 (0.028)	0.0078 (0.029)	0.0026 (0.021)	0.027 (0.022)	0.069 (0.044)
CLT16	0.012 (0.014)	-0.012 (0.012)	0.009 (0.014)	0.018 (0.011)	0.0017 (0.011)	-0.0060 (0.0098)	0.014 (0.011)	0.011 (0.023)
CLT19	-0.011 (0.027)	-0.062 (0.022)	-0.082 (0.028)	-0.047 (0.023)	-0.020 (0.022)	-0.026 (0.019)	0.043 (0.022)	-0.0019 (0.046)
NE	-0.206 (0.061)	-0.027 (0.056)	-0.131 (0.064)	-0.107 (0.051)	-0.151 (0.057)	-0.091 (0.044)	-0.104 (0.051)	-0.112 (0.089)
MA	-0.092 (0.051)	0.063 (0.040)	-0.052 (0.048)	-0.033 (0.040)	-0.140 (0.043)	-0.050 (0.033)	-0.092 (0.036)	-0.067 (0.074)

Table 4-5 *(continued)*

Variable	Males				Females			
	HOSP	MNOR	GULD	UNST	HOSP	MNOR	GULD	UNST
ENC	0.069 (0.077)	7.055 (0.033)	0.066 (0.034)	-0.0094 (0.043)	-0.062 (0.041)	0.072 (0.043)	0.060 (0.039)	-0.095 (0.049)
WNC	-0.012 (0.095)	-0.069 (0.050)	-0.094 (0.043)	-0.140 (0.051)	-0.173 (0.048)	-0.113 (0.064)	-0.112 (0.049)	-0.216 (0.060)
SA	-0.021 (0.088)	-0.010 (0.043)	-0.033 (0.035)	-0.080 (0.044)	-0.032 (0.045)	0.077 (0.054)	0.040 (0.042)	-0.051 (0.057)
ESC	0.022 (0.097)	-0.073 (0.051)	-0.085 (0.045)	-0.249 (0.057)	-0.051 (0.058)	-0.021 (0.071)	-0.002 (0.056)	-0.188 (0.065)
WSC	-0.010 (0.086)	0.020 (0.046)	-0.084 (0.038)	-0.180 (0.050)	-0.112 (0.050)	-0.013 (0.056)	0.004 (0.047)	-0.142 (0.058)
MT	-0.104 (0.147)	-0.131 (0.067)	-0.122 (0.054)	-0.097 (0.068)	-0.129 (0.069)	0.145 (0.098)	-0.031 (0.065)	-0.209 (0.081)
CONSTANT	0.307	0.751	0.657	0.918	0.456	0.676	0.671	1.075
	$R^2 = 0.37$ $F(33,306)$ $= 5.53$	$R^2 = 0.25$ $F(33,1593)$ $= 15.74$	$R^2 = 0.23$ $F(33,2715)$ $= 24.69$	$R^2 = 0.22$ $F(33,1514)$ $= 12.62$	$R^2 = 0.27$ $F(33,1280)$ $= 14.49$	$R^2 = 0.19$ $F(33,861)$ $= 6.28$	$R^2 = 0.09$ $F(33,1638)$ $= 5.20$	$R^2 = 0.15$ $F(33,876)$ $= 4.49$

Note: Figures in parentheses are standard errors.

especially important effects on wages in the manorial industries. This result supports previous research (Alexander 1974) using the same industry categories. By contrast, occupation-specific experience has essentially no impact on wages in the manorial industry; it does affect hospital and unstructured industry wages for reasons that are far from obvious.

Since most blacks in both the 1960 and 1970 samples were also born in the states of the Confederacy, it is appropriate to examine coefficients of BLACK and BC (for blacks born in the Confederate states) jointly. In 1960 blacks' hourly wages were considerably lower than whites; the differences were more pronounced for males than for females. Comparatively speaking, blacks were less disadvantaged in the hospital sector than in the reference industries. Black male guild workers earned about 28 percent less, other things being equal, than their white coworkers. Surprisingly, the black-white wage differentials remained fairly large in 1970; in some instances, they had widened since 1960. Differentials in the hospital sector were 14 percent for males and 15 percent for females. Especially for 1970, it is difficult to argue that the black-white wage differences reflect something other than discrimination; the regressions contain thirty-one variables besides the two identifying blacks.

Differences in wages between Spanish-surnamed persons and whites were greater on the whole in 1970 than in 1960; and hospitals, if anything, would appear to be more discriminatory than the reference industries. No consistent pattern is evident in the coefficients of foreign-birth variables FR1, FR2, and FR3.

Several patterns in the marital status and children variables also merit attention. These should be examined, however, in conjunction with results from the annual earnings variables; for this reason, and because the behavior of these variables is not crucial to this chapter, we do not discuss them explicity.[1][2]

Wage Decomposition Analysis

Although it is certainly possible to discern interindustry variations in variable means and estimated parameters, it is virtually impossible to make summary statements about variations in employee mix by industry type from tables 4-2 through 4-5, since there are so many employee characteristics variables in the regressions. However, the decomposition methodology we have described does permit such statements.

Table 4-6 presents the decomposition analysis. Column (1) gives the reference industry category being compared with hospitals. Hospital employees are always in the numerator. Thus the crude wage difference of 0.626, which involves a hospital-manorial comparison for males in 1960, means that hourly wages of male hospital workers were 62.6 percent of their manorial counterparts in 1960. The first and second rows in each couplet are based on equations 4.1 and 4.2, respectively. In every case, the two equations yield very similar results.

Table 4-6
Wage Decomposition Analysis: Hospital Workers' Wages and "Quality" as a Proportion of Reference Industry Workers' Wages and "Quality"

Reference Group (1)	Crude Wage Difference		"Pure" Wage Difference		"Quality" Difference	
	1960 (2)	1970 (3)	1960 (4)	1970 (5)	1960 (6)	1970 (7)
Males						
Manorial[a]	0.626	0.721	0.670	0.750	0.934	0.962
Manorial[b]	0.626	0.721	0.696	0.750	0.899	0.960
Guild[a]	0.779	0.863	0.805	0.809	0.968	1.067
Guild[b]	0.779	0.863	0.780	0.809	0.998	1.067
Unstructured[a]	0.825	1.028	0.861	0.930	0.959	1.106
Unstructured[b]	0.825	1.028	0.827	0.919	0.998	1.119
Females						
Manorial[a]	0.788	0.885	0.798	0.861	0.988	1.028
Manorial[b]	0.788	0.885	0.769	0.841	1.025	1.052
Guild[a]	1.089	1.123	1.031	1.004	1.052	1.119
Guild[b]	1.089	1.123	1.016	1.037	1.071	1.083
Unstructured[a]	1.046	1.114	1.014	0.995	1.029	1.120
Unstructured[b]	1.046	1.114	0.980	1.027	1.067	1.084

[a]Based on equation 4-1.
[b]Based on equation 4-2.

Examination of columns (2) and (3) confirms a result evident from the means in tables 4-2 and 4-3. The rank order of male hourly wages for the reference industry categories in both years is manorial, guild, and unstructured. Hourly wages of male manorial and guild industry workers exceeded those of male hospital employees in 1960 and 1970. By 1970, male hospital workers' wages slightly exceeded those in unstructured industries.

The patterns for females are somewhat different. In contrast to males, hourly wages in unstructured industries exceeded those for the guild workers, even in 1960. By 1970, female hospital employees' wages exceeded guild and unstructured wages by 12 and 11 percent, respectively.

Patterns in crude wage differentials uniformly reveal that hourly wages of hospital employees increased in relative terms during the decade of the 1960s, a result confirming previous research by Feldstein (1971), Fuchs, (1976), and Feldstein and Taylor (1977). Beyond the crude wage differentials, however, data in table 4-6 offer implications that are in sharp contrast to much of previous research.

Columns (4) and (5) show pure wage differentials by sex, year, and industry group. The most marked differences are between male hospital employees and

their counterparts in manorial industries. Holding numerous worker characteristics constant, hospitals in 1960 paid their male employees on the average
two-thirds as much as they would have earned in manorial industries. By 1970,
hospitals paid their male employees three-quarters as much.

In general, pure wage differentials are smaller for female employees. There
was approximate parity between hospital, guild, and unstructured industries in
both 1960 and 1970. However, hospital-manorial differentials were substantial,
even in 1970.

The persistence of long-standing pure wage differentials raises serious
questions about the utility of traditional neoclassical models of labor markets.
Neoclassical economic theory explains equilibrium (or persistent) differentials in
terms of working conditions, prestige, and related factors. Are we to attribute
long-standing variations in quality-adjusted wages to job-related amenities? It
seems unlikely that working in a hospital setting is seen by employees as that
much more pleasant or prestigious than other settings. The persistence of pure
wage differentials of the type reported in table 4-6 also makes it difficult to
argue for the philanthropic wage hypothesis. Hospitals seem not to be bestowing
any particular favors on their employees, at least gauged in terms of financial
compensation.

The quality differences in columns (6) and (7) reveal that the hospital work
force was, with one exception (male manorial workers in 1960), at least as
desirable as the work forces in the reference industries, and that quality of the
hospital work force rose relatively over the 1960s. With the exception of male
hospital-manorial differentials, the growth in hospital crude hourly wages,
relative to those in the reference industries, reflects increases in quality far more
than increases in pure wages.

This evidence implies that more plausible than the philanthropic wage
hypothesis is the view that improved third-party financing has encouraged
hospitals to upgrade their work forces. From the vantage point of policy, one
may wish to question whether upgrading is desirable; but surely, the method of
transferring income to hospital workers suggested by the philanthropic wage
hypothesis is even less desirable.[13] More rigorous empirical tests of the notion
that third-party reimbursement has a greater effect on work-force quality than
on pure wages are found in the next section.

Constructing State Means

The final stage of our census analysis uses the state rather than the individual as
the observational unit. Seven hypotheses pertinent to the state analysis were
presented in the introduction to this chapter. Regression analysis, using state
data, provides the basis for testing these hypotheses.

State means have been constructed from the 1960 and 1970 census data bases and estimated parameters for hospital employees (from tables 4-4 and 4-5) for these years. Information on reference industry groups plays no part in the state analysis. To elaborate on the method to be followed in this section, let

$w_{..}$ = the hospital wage for the entire United States

$w_{i.}$ = the crude hospital wage for state i

$\widetilde{w}_{i.}$ = the quality-adjusted wage in state i —assuming national wage-setting parameters and the state's skill mix

Thus for any state ,

$$\frac{w_{i.}}{w_{..}} = \frac{w_{i.}}{\widetilde{w}_{i.}} \cdot \frac{\widetilde{w}_{i.}}{w_{..}} \tag{4.3}$$

In equation 4.3 $\widetilde{w}_{i.}/w_{..}$ represents the quality of state i's hospital work force; $w_{i.}/\widetilde{w}_{i.}$ is the quality-adjusted wage. One could have written the quality term without $w_{..}$, but use of $w_{..}$ normalizes the quality index about 1.0. Separate versions of equation 4.3 have been developed for male and female hospital employees and for 1960 and 1970. Although equation 4.3 is cast in terms of wages, the formula is equally applicable to earnings; state means of work-force quality and quality-adjusted earnings, based on parameter estimates from annual earnings regressions, have been calculated and are used as dependent variables, along with their wage counterparts, in this section's empirical analysis.

State Wage Equation Specification

As in the previous section, it is possible to specify a much more complete equation for 1970 than for 1960. For this reason, the 1970 specification and findings will receive greater emphasis. Data sources and detail on state variable construction are presented in appendix G. A few regressions are based on annual earnings rather than hourly wages. The method described by equations 4.1 through 4.3 applies to earnings as well.

In the following tables, type W regressions use $w_i/\widetilde{w}_i$ or pure wage differentials as the dependent variable; type Q regressions have the quality index $\widetilde{w}_i/w_{..}$ as the dependent variable. The dependent variable in the Q regressions is conditional on an exogenous quality-adjusted wage, $w_{i.}/\widetilde{w}_{i.}$ = QWAGE, in the state regression analysis. With QWAGE an explanatory variable and the work-force quality index the dependent variable, one can test the hypothesis that the "own" quality-adjusted wage effect on quality is negative—that is, in states where hospitals pay higher quality-adjusted wages, do hospitals, other things being equal, employ a lower quality work force? Since QWAGE is itself a dependent variable, the model is recursive with factors affecting work force quality via their effects on the quality-adjusted wage.

Separate regressions are estimated for males and females (M and F in tables 4-7 through 4-9). Explanatory variables fall into three categories: (1) demand for hospital product; (2) general labor market conditions in the state; and (3) unionization. All monetarily expressed variables are deflated by a state price index in 1960 dollars. Observations are weighted by state population.

Assuming that what one observes in a cross section is a competitive equilibrium with a horizontal long-run labor supply curve (as seen in chapter 2), it is appropriate to include *product demand variables* in equations for the quantity and/or quality of labor demanded, but not in an equation with the pure quality-adjusted wage as the dependent variable. Under conditions of temporary and excess demand disequilibrium, an upward-sloping long-run supply curve, and/or market imperfections (for example, monopsony), it is appropriate to include product demand variables as explanatory variables in a quality-adjusted wage equation.

Among demand variables, the role of third-party reimbursement commands the greatest interest from the standpoint of public policy. Two *alternative* measures of the depth of private insurance coverage are included, INS1 and INS2, representing depth of total and hospital insurance coverage in the state, respectively. The variables have been constructed from verified health premium information from the Center for Health Administration Studies' (CHAS) 1971 survey of health care utilization and expenditures. These variables are described in appendix F and discussed in detail in Sloan and Steinwald (forthcoming, 1980). REIM is the proportion of expenditures on hospital services in the state paid by third-party payors, both private and public. This variable, applied to SMSAs rather than states, was used in chapter 3. Since private insurance is an important component of REIM, REIM enters as an alternative to INS1 or INS2. In specifications containing INS1 or INS2, the variable MCAID—state and local expenditures on medical assistance (primarily Medicaid) per capita population— is included as an explanatory variable. The INS1, INS2, and MCAID variables appear only in 1970 state regressions.

Other demand variables, all defined for the state, are: personal per capita income (INC); density—population per square mile (DENS); physicians per 1,000 population (MD); and two health status measures, LIM and HLTH. Both LIM and HLTH are based on synthetic estimates of disability developed by the National Center for Health Statistics. The variable LIM, based on synthetic estimates for 1962-1964 and used in the cross-sectional analysis for 1960, is the estimated percentage of the state population with activity limitations due to chronic conditions. HLTH, used in the 1970 analysis, is based on the estimated percentages of persons in the state falling into these mutually exclusive groups: (1) not limited in activity; (2) not limited in major activity but otherwise limited; (3) limited in amount or kind of major activity performed; and

(4) unable to carry on major activity. These percentages are weighted by data for the entire United States on mean number of hospital days per annum of persons in each of the four activity limitation categories. Data used to construct HLTH correspond to 1969-1971.

Local labor market conditions are represented by the mean manufacturing wage (MW) and unemployment rate (UN) for the state. MW and UN are expected to have positive and negative effects on quality-adjusted wages, respectively. It is worth recalling, however, that UN had a positive effect on wages in the last chapter for reasons we cannot explain.

The 1960 quality-adjusted wage regressions include MWAGE, which equals the state minimum wage applicable to hospital employees if a law existed in 1960.[14] Of the forty-nine states in the coterminous United States (including the District of Columbia), thirteen had such legislation in 1960; in at least half of these cases, the state had passed the minimum wage law in 1958, 1959, or 1960. Thus it is quite likely that MWAGE would have had no meaningful effect by 1960, especially since the dependent variable is based on annual earnings for 1959. As noted in chapter 3, a minimum wage could have a negative impact on hospital wages if hospital employees were specifically excluded. But hospital employees were excluded too infrequently to permit us to specify two minimum wage variables, one when they were included and another when they were not.

Finally, three *unionization* measures are included in the 1970 analysis: the proportion of short-term general hospitals in the state as of 1970 with collective bargaining agreements (CBARG); the proportion of such hospitals receiving a formal request for union representation during the year before the 1970 American Hospital Association survey (CBREQ); and the proportion of such hospitals experiencing a work stoppage or strike action during this period (STR). Coefficients on all three variables are expected to be positive. The CBREQ variable represents a threat effect.[15]

All variables (including the dependent variables) except the minimum wage and union variables, which frequently take on zero values, are in log form. Thus the vast majority of coefficients are elasticities.

Empirical Results of State
Cross-Sectional Analysis

Tables 4-7 through 4-9 present empirical results of the state cross-sectional regression analysis. Tables 4-8 and 4-9 differ in their specifications of insurance variables. In general the 1970 analysis yielded more plausible results. Empirical evidence on each of the seven hypotheses is discussed in turn.

Hypothesis 1 states that work-force quality is a normal good. As such, quality should respond positively to increased third-party coverage and rising real incomes in the state. Type Q regressions in the tables have work-force

Table 4-7
1960 State Census Regressions

Sex	Type[a]	CONS	INC	REIM	LIM	MD	DENS	MW	MWAGE	UN	QWAGE	
							Explanatory Variables					
M	Q	-0.50	0.023 (0.109)	0.0092 (0.0047)	-0.007 (0.094)	-0.042 (0.050)	-0.009 (0.014)				0.003 (0.079)	$R^2 = 0.16$ $F_{(6, 43)} = 1.4$
M	W	-4.48	0.78* (0.29)	-0.042 (0.098)	0.151 (0.193)	-0.42* (0.16)	0.023 (0.033)	0.074 (0.242)	0.063 (0.062)	0.14 (0.10)		$R^2 = 0.45$ $F_{(8, 41)} = 4.2$
F	Q	-0.93	0.063 (0.058)	-0.020 (0.029)	0.050 (0.059)	0.10* (0.03)	-0.013 (0.008)				0.043 (0.066)	$R^2 = 0.46$ $F_{(6, 41)} = 5.7$
F	W	-2.83	0.354 (0.209)	0.072 (0.066)	0.022 (0.139)	-0.09 (0.10)	-0.013 (0.021)	-0.003 (0.004)	-0.286 (0.173)	0.21* (0.06)		$R^2 = 0.30$ $F_{(8, 41)} = 2.1$

Note: Figures in parentheses are standard errors.

[a]Q = quality regression; W = quality-adjusted wage regression. The dependent variables for all regressions in this table are based on the micro wage regressions presented earlier in this chapter.

*Statistically significant at the 1 percent level (two-tail test).

Table 4-8
1970 State Census Regressions: First Specification

Sex	Type[a]	W or E[b]	CONS	INC	INS1	INS2	MCAID	HLTH	MD	DENS	MW	UN	CBARG	CBREQ	STR	QWAGE	
M	Q	W	-1.19	0.16 (0.13)	0.0005 (0.0391)		0.0006 (0.0118)	-0.13 (0.12)	0.0007 (0.0482)	-0.016 (0.009)				-0.0025 (0.228)	1.65* (0.48)	-0.072 (0.093)	$R^2 = 0.19$ $F_{(7, 42)} = 1.4$
M	W	W	-0.13								0.11 (0.09)	-0.037* (0.013)	0.16 (0.11)				$R^2 = 0.36$ $F_{(5, 44)} = 4.9$
M	W	W	-2.03	0.34 (0.22)	-0.062 (0.063)		-0.015 (0.020)	-0.11 (0.19)	-0.081 (0.088)	0.018 (0.017)	-0.002 (0.121)	-0.039** (0.015)	0.28** (0.13)	-0.37 (0.33)	1.44* (0.51)		$R^2 = 0.48$ $F_{(11, 38)} = 3.2$
M	W	W	-2.15	0.34 (0.22)		-0.049 (0.052)	-0.013 (0.020)	-0.12 (0.19)	-0.077 (0.087)	0.019 (0.017)	-0.011 (0.123)	-0.037** (0.015)	0.28** (0.13)	-0.36 (0.33)	1.40* (0.51)		$R^2 = 0.48$ $F_{(11, 38)} = 3.2$
M	W	E	-2.45	0.37 (0.34)	-0.029 (0.093)		-0.030 (0.030)	-0.19 (0.28)	-0.090 (0.129)	0.002 (0.025)	0.006 (0.176)	-0.029 (0.022)	0.44** (0.19)	-0.81 (0.48)	1.86** (0.76)		$R^2 = 0.36$ $F_{(11, 38)} = 1.9$
F	Q	W	-0.25	0.03 (0.05)	-0.078* (0.017)		-0.003 (0.056)	-0.16* (0.05)	0.084* (0.020)	0.002 (0.037)						-0.11 (0.06)	$R^2 = 0.80$ $F_{(7, 42)} = 23.5$
F	W	W	-0.07								0.006 (0.061)	-0.005 (0.009)	0.13 (0.08)	0.16 (0.16)	1.19* (0.34)		$R^2 = 0.52$ $F_{(5, 44)} = 9.5$
F	W	W	-0.68	0.11 (0.13)	-0.083** (0.041)		-0.010 (0.013)	0.021 (0.125)	0.007 (0.055)	0.021** (0.010)	0.007 (0.079)	-0.010 (0.010)	0.18** (0.09)	-0.18 (0.21)	1.19* (0.34)		$R^2 = 0.65$ $F_{(11, 38)} = 6.5$

Note: Figures in parentheses are standard errors.

[a] Q = quality regression; W = quality-adjusted wage regression.

[b] W = dependent variable based on wage regressions presented in this chapter; E = dependent variable based on annual earnings (micro) regressions presented in appendix F.

*Statistically significant at the 1 percent level (two-tail test); **Statistically significant at the 5 percent level (two-tail test).

Table 4-9
1970 State Census Regressions: Second Specification

Sex	Type[a]	W or E[b]	CONS	INC	REIM	HLTH	MD	DENS	MW	UN	CBARG	CBREQ	STR	QWAGE	
							Explanatory Variables								
M	Q	W	-0.99	0.14 (0.13)	-0.016 (0.088)	-0.15 (0.12)	0.020 (0.040)	-0.014 (0.008)						-0.06 (0.10)	$R^2 = 0.18$ $F_{(6, 43)} = 1.6$
M	W	W	-4.29	0.38 (0.24)	0.26 (0.17)	0.004 (0.221)	-0.081 (0.085)	0.009 (0.019)	-0.042 (0.137)	-0.043** (0.016)	0.22 (0.14)	-0.44 (0.37)	1.00 (0.59)		$R^2 = 0.50$ $F_{(10, 39)} = 3.9$
M	W	E	-3.96	0.44 (0.32)	0.14 (0.22)	-0.057 (0.290)	-0.13 (0.11)	0.009 (0.026)	0.004 (0.180)	-0.032 (0.021)	0.37** (0.19)	-0.82 (0.48)	1.56** (0.79)		$R^2 = 0.35$ $F_{(10, 39)} = 2.1$
F	Q	W	-0.55	0.017 (0.058)	-0.014 (0.043)	-0.16** (0.07)	0.11* (0.02)	-0.0065 (0.0040)						-0.05 (0.07)	$R^2 = 0.69$ $F_{(6, 43)} = 15.9$
F	W	W	-1.64	0.124 (0.130)	0.054 (0.093)	0.084 (0.129)	0.032 (0.048)	0.015 (0.010)	0.021 (0.078)	-0.014 (0.009)	0.17** (0.08)	-0.23 (0.21)	0.98* (0.34)		$R^2 = 0.62$ $F_{(10, 39)} = 8.4$

Note: Figures in parentheses are standard errors.

[a]Q = quality regression; W = quality-adjusted wage regression.

[b]W = dependent variable based on wage regressions presented in this chapter; E = dependent variable based on annual earnings (micro) regressions presented in appendix F.

*Statistically significant at the 1 percent level (two-tail test); **Statistically significant at the 5 percent level (two-tail test).

quality as the dependent variable. Only in one of the two 1960 regressions (table 4-7) does the parameter estimate of the fraction of hospital expenditures covered by third-party sources (REIM) have the expected positive sign; REIM demonstrates an implausible negative effect on work-force quality in the two 1970 Q regressions in which the variable enters. Similar results are obtained when INS1 or INS2 represent private insurance (see table 4-8). The coefficients on the per capita income variable, although consistently positive, are frequently less than their standard errors. Income and third-party coverage for hospital services rose markedly during the 1960s, and table 4-6 indicates an upgrading of work-force quality relative to the reference industries. But although time series evidence is suggestive, a similar pattern is not evident from single cross sections. The fraction of hospital expenses covered (REIM) performed much better in last chapter's time series cross-sectional analysis. A study by Davis (1973) also showed reimbursement to have a stronger impact in a time series cross-sectional analysis than in research on single cross sections. Considering table 4-6 as well as tables 4-7 through 4-9, there is evidence both for and against hypothesis 1. Judging from trends alone (table 4-6), it would appear that the growth in personal income and insurance coverage contributed to the upgrading of the hospital labor force. We are, however, unable to find a relationship in our cross-sectional regression analysis with states as the observational units.

According to hypothesis 2, the "own" quality-adjusted wage effect on demand for work-force quality is negative—that is, hospitals in states in which quality-adjusted wages are higher should purchase lower quality labor. The negative signs of the QWAGE coefficients in the 1970 regressions are consistent with the hypothesis; but their magnitudes imply elasticities of 0.11 or less, and, with one exception, the associated standard errors are large. The positive signs in QWAGE in the 1960 analysis (table 4-7) are inconsistent with hypothesis 2. Thus our evidence in favor of hypothesis 2—namely, that the quality-adjusted wage exerts a negative influence on hospital demand for work-force quality—is weak at best.

According to hypothesis 3, quality-adjusted wages are higher in states with substantial amounts of hospital union activity, as measured by the three union variables. The major part of this hypothesis is strongly confirmed by the state cross-sectional analysis. The CBARG coefficients imply that pure wages are on the average 13 to 28 percent higher in hospitals with collective bargaining agreements. These estimates are somewhat higher than the 3 to 18 percent range obtained in the preceding chapter's analysis of Bureau of Labor Statistics data. According to unpublished AHA data used to construct our union variables in this and subsequent chapters, as of 1970, 19 percent of hospitals had collective bargaining agreements. The impact of CBARG on quality-adjusted annual earnings of males is considerably higher, 44 and 37 percent (in regression 5, table 4-8; and regression 3, table 4-9 respectively), than on quality-adjusted hourly wages. This result may in part be because of a possible tendency for unionization to decrease the proportion of part-time employees.

The STR parameter estimates imply that quality-adjusted wages are over twice as high in hospitals in which a strike or other work stoppage occurred in the previous year. These estimates undoubtedly attribute too much power to collective action. In 1969-1970, only 3.2 percent of short-term general hospitals experienced a work stoppage, not a meaningful proportion of U.S. hospitals. Yet in combination with the results on CBARG, the STR results suggest that union activities are an important source of hospital wage inflation.

With one exception, the coefficients on the union recognition request variable CBREQ are negative. This result implies that the threat effect, if anything, is negligible in a hospital context. Wages rise after the union is introduced in a hospital, not in anticipation of its possible introduction. Overall, hypothesis 3, which states that union activity raises the quality-adjusted wage, is strongly confirmed.

Hypothesis 4 maintains that minimum wages raise quality-adjusted wages. Since by 1970 the federal minimum wage law applied to hospitals, the hypothesis can only be tested with reference to the 1960 state cross-section. In the two regressions in which MWAGE enters in table 4-7, the MWAGE parameter estimate is positive only once. On the basis of table 4-7, hypothesis 4 should be rejected.

However, results consistent with hypothesis 4 were reported in chapter 3, where minimum wage elasticities ranged as high as 0.15. There are a number of possible explanations for the difference. First, and most important, many state minimum wage laws were too recent to have had a discernible impact by 1960. Second, in chapter 3, the dependent wage variable did not hold work-force quality constant. One possible effect of such laws is to encourage covered employers to select higher quality employees. But since the occupations analyzed in chapter 3 were quite specific, it is doubtful that there was substantial room for quality variations within occupations. Hence, on balance, we believe hypothesis 4 can be accepted, but not on the basis of this chapter's empirical analysis.

According to hypothesis 5, quality-adjusted wages partly reflect the tightness of state labor markets as measured by the state unemployment rate. The unemployment rate (UN) demonstrates the anticipated negative impact in the 1970 regressions. In the male employee regressions, the coefficients tend to be statistically significant with associated elasticities in the 0.03 to 0.04 range; though negative, the coefficients are insignificant in the female regressions. The UN coefficients are implausibly positive in the 1960 regressions. Unfortunately, the BLS did not provide a state unemployment series as early as 1960; therefore, data for UN came from the 1960 census. It is doubtful that the UN measure, based on data for a single 1960 census reference week, is necessarily indicative of labor market tightness during 1959-1960. Thus the evidence in this chapter leads to a standoff on hypothesis 5. Before reaching any overal conclusions on this issue, we should consider evidence presented in the following chapter.

According to hypothesis 6, labor markets take a long time to clear. Allowing for disequilibrium (albeit a temporary one), there is clearly a role for product demand variables in state cross-sectional analysis of quality-adjusted wages. Among product demand variables, per capita income has the most notable effect. In male regressions, INC parameter estimates are consistently positive with associated t ratios always exceeding one; elasticities range from 0.34 to 0.38 with quality-adjusted wages as the dependent variable. INC elasticities from regressions with quality-adjusted earnings as the dependent variable are slightly higher. For reasons difficult to understand, the INC parameter estimates are lower and less significant in the female regressions in both years. As noted in chapter 2, there is a role for demand variables in equilibrium as long as the supply of labor curve has a positive slope. To fully attribute the results on INC to disequilibrium, we need evidence on hypothesis 7.

To test hypothesis 7—that quality-adjusted wages are highest in states in which the 1965-1970 growth of hospital work force was most rapid—a variable representing hospital work-force growth was included in regressions not shown. This variable showed no effect on quality-adjusted wages. Thus there is some reason to attribute the results on INC in our discussion of hypothesis 6 to something other than disequilibrium per se.

Conclusions and Implications

In an article titled "The Earnings of Allied Health Personnel—Are Health Workers Underpaid?" Fuchs (1976) concluded that, relative to workers with comparable attributes in other nonfarm industries, health service industry workers are not underpaid.

More specifically, Fuchs found that "females [in health settings] do better than males, hospital workers do better than workers in other health settings . . . and the data also indicate that this equality has been achieved since 1959" (p. 425).

Although this chapter employs the same basic data source as the Fuchs article, there are methodological differences between the two studies. First, Fuchs standardized work-force composition on four characteristics; we have used a far more detailed set of characteristics. Second, Fuchs compared health workers in general and hospital workers in particular to a composite category of all nonfarm industries; we have compared hospital employees with those in three more homogeneous reference industries. As has been shown, there is substantial interindustry variation in the growth in real wages. To answer the question Fuchs posed in the title of his article, one must add, "underpaid relative to whom?" Third, our study analyzes growth in work-force "quality" and in "pure" wages; Fuchs examined only the latter. As in other chapters, we have attempted to *explain* observed variations in hospital wages as well as presenting pertinent descriptive information.

Consistent with Fuchs' findings, evidence presented in this chapter indicates that wages of hospital workers rose relative to other nonfarm industries during the 1960s. This is true of both unadjusted wages in particular and, to a lesser extent, quality-adjusted wages that hold characteristics of hospital and reference industry employees constant. Using tabulations to adjust for work-force characteristics, Fuchs found that by the end of the 1960s, adjusted hourly earnings of white and nonwhite male hospital employees were, respectively, 0.84 and 0.88 of their counterparts in nonfarm industries. For white and nonwhite females, corresponding ratios were 1.02 and 1.04. Fuchs' estimates for males fall in the midrange of the estimates presented in this chapter. His female estimates, though comparable to this chapter's estimates of pure wage differences between hospitals and guild and unstructured industries, are far higher than the ratio of wages of female hospital employees to their counterparts in the manorial industries.

Are hospital workers underpaid? Judging from this chapter's estimates, it is clear that they are not overpaid on average. Relative to male employees in the reference industries, male hospital employees were still underpaid in 1970. Relative wages of female hospital employees were more favorable, although they earned about 15 percent less than female manorial industry workers.

Far more important than the increase in quality-adjusted wages of hospital workers during the 1960s was the upgrading of the hospital work force during this period. The Fuchs study has nothing to say about this phenomenon. Comparing 1960 and 1970, one may reasonably infer that this upgrading is at least partly attributable to general prosperity of the 1960s and to increased third-party reimbursement. However, the generally weak performance of the reimbursement variables in the previous section is sufficient reason to be cautious about making too strong a statement about the role of insurance.

In view of this chapter's evidence, and Fuchs' for that matter, it is very difficult to call hospital administrators "philanthropists." They understandably may have converted improved patient ability to pay into a more desirable, higher quality work force, even though the link between financing and work-force quality from our state regression analysis is weak. This interpretation of events makes more theoretical sense than Feldstein's argument, in any case. If hospitals offered employees above-normal wages, they would most likely face a perpetual queue of job seekers outside the doors of their personnel offices. There would be more than a minor temptation to select the most qualified workers from the queue. From the vantage point of the third party, it is probably far easier to justify high wages as "reasonable" if they result in a more productive labor force than if they represent pure philanthropy.

Of the seven hypotheses tested in the last section, the strongest results relate to the effect of union activity on the quality-adjusted wage. Clearly, unionization matters; and further expansion of such activity will most likely lead to increased growth in real hospital wages. Of course, other forces, including hospital regulation, may operate in the opposite direction. The next chapter focuses on regulatory impacts on wages.

Notes

1. Feldstein (1971), Fuchs (1976), and Feldstein and Taylor (1977).
2. Feldstein (1971), and Feldstein and Taylor (1977).
3. Unfortunately (at least to our knowledge) there is no other empirical evidence specifically linking turnover of hospital employees to wages. For a comprehensive general review of the turnover literature, see Price (1977).
4. Job satisfaction studies are reviewed by Jelinek and Dennis (1976).
5. See Weiss (1966), Wachtel and Betsey (1972), Thurow (1975), and chapter 2.
6. Kerr (1954), Doeringer and Piore (1971).
7. Annual earnings regressions have also been estimated. See appendix F.
8. See appendix A for a description.
9. The marriage variables may also pick up variations in effort on the job, especially for males. See Becker (mimeo).
10. The BC variable stems from Weiss (1970), blacks born (and raised) in the South may have had worse schooling than blacks from other regions. Race-ethnicity variables account for discrimination, both past and present.
11. Our experience variables, based on an algorithm previously employed by Hanoch (1965), Mincer (1974), and Schultz (1975), is defined as the difference in years between respondent's age and age when she/he is assumed to have entered the labor force:

Assumed age of entry into labor force	Schooling grade completed
10	<5
14	5-7
16	8
18	9-11
20	12
23	13-15
26	16
28	17-20

12. Earnings regressions, based on individual observations from the U.S. censuses, are presented in appendix F.

13. Assuming the hospital sector faces an upward-sloping supply curve of labor, at least for certain specialized occupations, an outward shift in the demand curve resulting in an increase in equilibrium wages will yield rents to inframarginal workers.

14. Given the extension of the Fair Labor Standards Act to hospital employees in 1967, there was no meaningful interstate variation to observe in a single cross section by 1970.

15. For a conceptual analysis of threat effects, see Rosen (1969).

5

Reimbursement and Regulatory Effects on Mean Annual Earnings of Hospital Employees

Introduction

This is the first of two chapters emphasizing hospital wage determination in the 1970s. Whereas the major public policy development affecting hospitals during the 1960s was the enactment of Medicare and Medicaid, the focus of much government attention in the hospital sphere during the 1970s has been on cost containment by means of regulation. Many of the regulatory efforts have been combined with third-party reimbursement mechanisms.

Recent forms of hospital regulation fall into three general categories: capital expenditures-facilities regulation; revenue-cost regulation; and utilization review. Prominent examples of the first category are:

1. State certificate-of-need (CON) laws, which mandate state-designated agencies to regulate the expansion and/or modernization of hospital plants as well as, in some cases, the provision of new hospital services.
2. The P.L. 92-603, Section 1122 Review Program, in which the states, as voluntary participants, use the reimbursement mechanisms of Social Security Act programs (the most important of which are Medicare and Medicaid) as a regulatory tool. Approval by state-designated planning agencies of hospital capital expenditures exceeding $100,000, changes in bed size, and/or changes in services offered is required as a precondition for full reimbursement.
3. Requirements of some Blue Cross plans for hospitals, to receive full reimbursement for services delivered to Blue Cross subscribers, to obtain approval from health planning agencies for certain cost-increasing capital expenditures.

Among the most important forms of revenue-cost regulation have been the Nixon Administration's Economic Stabilization Program (ESP); prospective reimbursement (PR) programs of several states and some Blue Cross plans; and regulatory restrictions under Medicare and Medicaid. Utilization review (UR) encompasses state Medicaid and Blue Cross programs, as well as the more recent Professional Standards Review Organization (PSRO) program instituted under P.L. 92-603, but not implemented on a widespread basis until the mid-1970s. The UR programs tend to have both cost containment and quality assurance objectives.

In contrast to market solutions that fundamentally rely on incentives, regulation offers the appeal of immediate solutions to perceived problems in the hospital sector. Laws can be written and regulations promulgated which get to the heart of the problem. Market approaches seem indirect; responses are slow; and, ultimately, they appear to aid provider-producer-investors, if anyone, and hence are objectionable on distributional grounds.

Despite these purported advantages, there is a growing belief that regulation may have been oversold. Even though regulation is directly aimed at one set of outcomes, there may be unanticipated side effects on the part of firms in the regulated industry. Rapid responses to regulation are often hindered by the litigation process, which occupies the energies of all parties. And because the provider-producer-investor has political and financial resources, regulatory agencies are subject to "capture."[1]

This chapter's data base consists of a time series of cross sections of 1,228 nonfederal, short-term general hospitals over six years, 1970 through 1975. Thus this chapter focuses on wage-setting decisions of a large cohort of U.S. hospitals. Another study by us[2] makes greater use of these data, but does not examine wage setting as such. Pertinent results from that study are reported here and contrasted with this chapter's findings.

The dependent variable in this chapter encompasses an element of skill mix as well as variations in the skill- or quality-adjusted wage. American Hospital Association (AHA) data allow one to construct mean annual earnings per hospital employee by dividing the total payroll by the number of full-time equivalent personnel employed by the hospital. The resulting earnings measure has been refined for this study by excluding employed physicians, physician trainees, RNs, and LPNs from both the payroll numerator and the full-time equivalent denominator. To exclude RNs and LPNs, we use wage measures developed from other sources. We refer to the dependent variable as "other employees' earnings" because the aforementioned occupations have been excluded. That our dependent variable encompasses some skill mix as well as pure wage variation is important and merits consideration at the outset.

We first examine the two potential effects of regulation on pure wages. Wage controls could suppress hospital wages directly. In the competitive labor market of textbooks, all hospital employees would quit, obtaining jobs in different industries. A large outflow might depress other wages somewhat, thus tempering the exodus. If all labor markets were subject to such controls, as under much of ESP, hospital employees would not have an incentive to move; but hospitals seeking additional workers because of an outward shift in the demand curve for their products would experience difficulties in hiring. If the hospitals faced an upward-sloping supply curve (that is, if they possessed a degree of monopsony power), controls would not cause massive terminations; but with outward shifting product demand curves, excess demand for hospital labor would arise. Few if any economists would maintain that employees face flat labor supply curves in the short run because of the transactions costs they face in changing jobs. Furthermore, at least for a while, employees are likely to find it best to wait out controls, lest they be lifted soon after the job change. Hence, under a variety of assumptions, there are conceptual reasons for expecting that controls can depress wages.

Most forms of regulation, however, are related more directly to the hospital's revenue and/or input use than to actual wages paid to employees. These programs potentially affect pure wages via derived demand. As noted previously exogenous forces on the demand side have no impact on wages in long-run competitive equilibrium as long as the labor supply curve is horizontal, but they do matter in imperfectly competitive labor markets or under conditions of temporary disequilibrium. In earlier chapters, we have found that the demand side plays a role in hospital wage setting. Hence, product demand-oriented controls should influence pure wages. When the wage series reflects skill mix as well as pure wage variations, impacts of regulation operating via the derived demand route should be more evident than when the skill-mix influence has been purged from the wage or earnings series. If, for example, a form of regulation inhibits the growth of sophisticated hospital services, employment of skilled personnel should be retarded as well.

While introductory statements generally dramatize the importance of the topic to be investigated, in this instance, we must reiterate that the growth in hospital wages has not been great in real terms during the 1970s. Calculations using this chapter's earnings measure indicate that over 1970-1975, the overall growth was 4.9 percent in real terms.[3] As shown in the first row of table 5-1, real mean annual earnings actually fell during 1973 and 1974. These patterns are consistent with evidence from other sources reported in chapters 1, 3, and 6.

Table 5-1
Other Employees' Earnings—National Trends, 1970-1975

	1970	1971	1972	1973	1974	1975	Grand Mean
Other Employees' Earnings deflated ($)	5,687	5,944	6,169	5,990	5,725	5,964	5,913
annual growth (%)		4.5	3.8	−2.9	−4.4	−4.2	
Other Employees' Earnings undeflated ($)	5,417	5,722	6,382	6,571	6,872	7,746	6,448
annual growth (%)		5.6	11.5	3.0	4.6	12.7	
AHA Earnings Series[a] undeflated ($)	5,921	6,529	7,051	7,368	7,787	8,635	7,220[b]
annual growth (%)		10.3	8.0	4.5	5.7	10.9	

[a]From AHA (1976), p. xii.

[b]The grand mean is unavailable from the AHA (1976) source. We have simply taken the average of the annual means in this row.

Two undeflated series are also presented in table 5-1. The second row comes from our data base and uses our earnings measure. For comparison purposes, an undeflated earnings series published by the AHA is presented in the third row. The AHA's undeflated series is higher than ours although growth rates over the 1970-1975 period are reasonably close (43 versus 46 percent for the AHA). Probably the most important reason for the discrepancy is our exclusion of the employee categories listed earlier, which are included in the AHA's series.

Table 5-2 shows trends in our earnings variable by census division. Although hospital employees in the Pacific census division had the highest earnings in 1975, the growth in real earnings over 1970-1975 was far less than for the other census divisions. Highest rates of (real) earnings inflation were in the two North Central and the Mountain census divisions.

The next section presents a very concise review of institutional aspects of hospital regulation, as well as some empirical results from past studies. The third section describes data, variable definitions, and model specification. In the fourth section, regression results are presented and discussed. Finally, conclusions and policy implications are examined.

Regulating the Hospital: Description and Empirical Evidence

Capital-Facilities Regulation

Capital-facilities regulation finds its rationale in "Roemer's law," which states that hospital beds generate their own demand.[4] This rationale reflects a concern that overinvestment in beds and other facilities leads to excess capacity,[5] which in turn must be supported by the public through third-party reimbursement; and a distributional concern of planners that capital expenditures are not made in areas where they are most needed. Advocates of this form of regulation expect that by curbing capital expenditures and specific facilities and services, the growth in hospital labor as well as nonlabor inputs will be reduced, both in raw numbers and in technical sophistication. Certificate-of-need (CON) laws, in particular, were given an impetus in 1974 with the passage by Congress of the National Health Planning and Resources Development Act, P.L. 94-641, which requires all states to adopt a CON program.[6]

As of the mid-1970s, most states had enacted CON laws and had also begun participating in the P.L. 92-603 Section 1122 review program.[7] Although Section 1122 programs are uniform among participating states, there is substantial interstate variation in CON in terms of comprehensiveness, thresholds for review, and review and appeals procedures. Coverage generally extends to hospitals and nursing homes but not to doctors' offices. Many state laws require detailed surveillance of health services, even when substantial capital expenditures are not involved. In these states, the appropriate agency must approve any

Table 5-2
Other Employees' Earnings—Trends by Census Division, 1970-1975

Census Division	1970	Deflated Dollars (Growth Percent Annual)					Growth 1970-1975 (%)
		1971	1972	1973	1974	1975	
New England	5,268	5,438 (3.2)	5,967 (9.7)	5,463 (-8.4)	5,330 (-2.4)	5,552 (4.2)	5.4
Mid-Atlantic	5,495	5,957 (8.4)	6,135 (3.0)	5,878 (-4.2)	5,617 (-4.4)	5,834 (3.9)	6.2
East North Central	5,564	5,934 (6.6)	6,053 (2.0)	5,907 (-2.4)	5,624 (-4.8)	6,038 (7.4)	8.5
West North Central	5,716	6,036 (5.6)	6,292 (4.2)	6,104 (-3.0)	5,967 (-2.2)	6,193 (3.8)	8.3
South Atlantic	4,967	5,083 (2.3)	5,474 (7.7)	5,400 (-1.4)	5,296 (-1.9)	5,334 (0.7)	7.4
East South Central	5,438	5,463 (0.5)	5,852 (7.1)	5,789 (-1.1)	5,435 (-6.1)	5,708 (5.0)	5.0
West South Central	5,135	5,375 (4.7)	5,590 (4.0)	5,411 (-3.2)	5,044 (-6.8)	5,334 (5.7)	3.9
Mountain	5,421	5,671 (4.6)	6,178 (8.9)	5,836 (-5.5)	5,439 (-6.8)	5,871 (7.9)	8.3
Pacific	6,596	6,760 (2.5)	6,957 (2.9)	6,749 (-3.0)	6,318 (-6.4)	6,376 (0.9)	-3.3

Note: Annual percentage rates of growth are given in parentheses.

significant change in special services offered. CON is a reactive form of regulation. The regulated institution rather than the agency takes the initiative in proposing a particular capital expenditure. Hospital decertification is now only in discussion stages.[8]

Past research on the effects on CON falls into three categories: single state-oriented studies; national studies of the structure of state CON programs and the process of planning-review-appeals; and regression studies. We confine our comments to highlights from the regression studies.[9]

Studies by Salkever and Bice (1976a, 1976b) and Hellinger (1976) are the best-known multivariate studies of capital-facilities regulation. To assess the impact of CON on hospital investment, Salkever and Bice used state data for the 1968-1972 period and found that CON reduced bed expansion, but increased plant assets per bed. The growth in plant assets per bed offset the reduction in bed expansion attributable to CON, leading to the conclusion that CON has no impact on total investment (change in plant assets). The authors gave two plausible reasons for their results. First, given strong pressures for capital expansion on hospital management, especially from the medical staff, a hospital facing a denial of its application for additional beds may "compensate" its physicians by installing facilities that either are not covered by the statute or, though covered, are more easily approved. Second, philanthropic funds not used to finance bed expansion may be made available to the hospital for other uses.

Of the fourteen types of facilities and services analyzed in the second part of their study, three types (extended care units, diagnostic radioscope, and intensive care units) showed statistically significant numerical increases attributable to CON, whereas a decrease would occur if CON review were effective. In the remaining eleven categories, CON showed no significant impacts. In another phase of their research, Salkever and Bice concluded that CON programs have not reduced hospital costs per capita population.

The Hellinger study, based on state data for 1972 and 1973, concluded that CON and Section 1122 programs have not significantly reduced hospital investment, even though uniformly negative signs pointed in this direction. Furthermore, Hellinger, like Lewin and Associates (1975), found some evidence to support the hypothesis that hospitals avoided any initial impact CON might have had by beginning projects before CON legislation was enacted. However, Hellinger's use of ordinary least squares (OLS) in regressions with a Koyck dynamic specification is highly objectionable on econometric grounds and probably resulted in serious biases in his estimated parameters.

Using the same data base as in this chapter, Sloan and Steinwald (forthcoming 1980) investigated the impacts of various forms of regulation, including CON, on both hospital costs and demand for labor and nonlabor inputs. Separate average hospital cost regressions were estimated for total and for labor expense, using adjusted patient days and admissions, alternatively, as denominators for the cost-dependent variables. The labor-expense regressions differed from those presented in this chapter in the following ways: first, the expense-dependent variables encompassed all types of hospital labor. Second, they reflected quantities of labor employed per unit of output as well as skill mix and skill-adjusted wages. Third, they incorporated an estimate of the dollar amount of fringe benefits. Several explanatory variables were specified to represent the potential influence of CON; the same ones are utilized in this chapter, and like other regulatory variables, are defined in the next section. In general, however, the estimated parameters associated with CON variables were positive, suggesting that on the whole, CON has raised labor costs (possibly a compensatory response to state regulation on the nonlabor input side). These results from our other study raise the question of whether a compensatory skill-mix effect will be evident from analysis of wage variations as well.

In contrast to CON, which gives the state the power to absolutely forbid unapproved capital expenditures, Section 1122 reviews and Blue Cross requirements for compliance with planning agency determination of need operate through the third-party reimbursement mechanism. Hospital expenditures attributable to unapproved capital projects are simply not reimbursed, and, presumably, the hospital has to secure funds to cover these expenses from other sources, including other third-party payors. Unlike CON, the clout of these programs is directly proportional to the fraction of hospital revenues from Medicare and Medicaid (Section 1122 programs) and Blue Cross (Blue Cross compliance programs). If these are unimportant revenue sources, the hospital may find it desirable to go ahead with a capital expenditure project without planning agency approval.

Sloan and Steinwald (forthcoming, 1980) found that Section 1122 programs had essentially zero effect in average expense regressions, incorporating labor as well as nonlabor costs; but they had a significantly positive effect on labor expense per adjusted patient day. Section 1122's effects on nonlabor inputs tended to be negative, but these negative effects were offset by positive coefficients in the labor demand regressions. The Blue Cross Planning Agency approval variable (BCPAA) demonstrated negative and significant effects on both total and labor expense per admission, and negative but insignificant effects in cost regressions with average costs per adjusted patient day denominators. The results on inputs were mixed. BCPAA had a significantly negative effect on bed expansion, but not on assets (or on assets per bed). The Blue Cross programs seem to have reduced hospital demand for RNs and LPNs, but stimulated demand for other employees.

Revenue-Cost Regulation

The only federal attempt to regulate hospital expenditures was the Economic Stabilization Program (ESP). Initially, beginning in August 1971, both wages and prices were controlled (although, inadvertently, not reimbursement of costs by third-party payors). In December 1972, regulations specific to institutional health care providers were issued. These limited the growth in annual revenue due to price increases to 6 percent; however, all price increases had to be cost justified. Limitations on increases in specific costs—5.5 percent for wages, 2.5 percent for nonlabor costs, and 1.7 for "new" technology—as well as limitations on increases in profit margins, could well have constrained many hospitals to service charge increases below the allowed 6 percent. As ESP progressed, unanticipated administrative problems and political considerations led to exceptions. Probably for the latter reason, wages of low-paid employees were exempted; but initially, the 5.5 percent overall restriction on wage increases applied, causing hardships for some hospitals that allowed wages of low-skilled employees to rise. Gradually, such inconsistencies were resolved; and later during the program hospitals were permitted to pass allowable cost increases through (to consumers and third party payors) on a dollar-for-dollar basis (Ginsburg 1976).

The most comprehensive general empirical evaluation of ESP's impact in the context of hospitals was done by Ginsburg (1976, 1978).[10] Using aggregate data for the nine U.S. census divisions for forty-four quarters (1963-1973) from the AHA's panel survey of hospitals, Ginsburg regressed a set of exogenous variables, including a dummy variable signifying the quarters during which ESP was in effect, on a number of variables related to hospital costs. Both static and dynamic versions of his model showed no significant effect, except on wages, in which case Ginsburg found that ESP had a significantly negative impact. In a static version, a decline in the ratio of labor to nonlabor inputs was attributable to ESP. His results on wages are not directly comparable to ours, however, since his wage variable was expressed in money rather than real terms (that is, his wage series was not deflated). Furthermore, his time series contained no post-ESP experience. That Ginsburg's time series only extended through 1973 is unfortunate since the ESP variable may have picked up other trends not related to ESP in the 1963-1973 decade's later years. More conclusive evidence could be obtained with a time series incorporating some post-ESP experience.

A more recent multivariate aggregate time series study of hospitals that includes some post-ESP data is by Taylor (1977). Like Ginsburg, Taylor based her analysis on the AHA's panel survey. As in our study, the dependent wage variables were expressed in real terms. Taylor found that real hospital wages were at least 4 percent below what they would have been in the absence of ESP. Furthermore, her labor demand regressions showed that ESP reduced hospital employment levels, but by less than 4 percent.

Another form of revenue-cost regulation is prospective reimbursement (PR), which has been defined by Dowling (1974) as "a method of paying hospitals in which (1) amounts or rates of payment are established in advance for the coming year, and (2) hospitals are paid these amounts or rates regardless of the costs they actually incur" (p. 163). In contradistinction to cost-based reimbursement in which (at least in principle) costs generate revenue, PR (again in principle) gives hospitals reason to be concerned with the cost implications of changes in quantity, quality, style of care, scope of services, and/or efficiency, because third-party payors under PR do not cover overruns. Uniformity among PR programs in the various states virtually ends with Dowling's definition. Programs differ according to: (1) whether they are mandatory or voluntary; (2) the use of a formula or budget review method for prospective rate setting; (3) the payors covered—for example, Medicaid, Blue Cross, private payors; (4) the payment unit—including patient day, case, specific services, total hospital or department budget; and (5) aspects of PR administration, including the locus of rate-setting authority.

One can safely conclude that voluntary systems—that is, those that give the hospital the option of participating in a PR experiment—are not likely to be effective as a general strategy for containing hospital cost growth. By contrast, the formula versus budget review distinction is an important one, and we develop separate PR variables in our empirical analysis for these two forms. Until recently, the only formula PR system was New York's, and because of the number of years and hospitals covered, the New York experience must dominate any current evaluation of formula PR, including ours. Under formula systems, the prospective rate is established by solving an equation consisting of variables pertaining to individual hospital characteristics (such as occupancy rate and prior cost experience), and factors external to the hospital (for example, general inflation rate). The formula is recomputed periodically, usually yearly, to arrive at a new prospective rate. This method involves relatively little direct interaction between hospitals and the rate-setting authority and is therefore less costly to administer and, although possibly more arbitrary, less likely to be redirected to the hospital's advantage.

Under budget PR systems, the hospital develops a budget for the prospective year which is reviewed by the PR authority. Items in the budget deemed unnecessary or excessive are eliminated or reduced. Hospitals are generally given the opportunity to negotiate and/or appeal budget-reducing decisions. Once the final budget has been approved, a payment rate is established that covers the hospital's budgeted costs. Because this method permits maximum recognition of individual hospital characteristics, hospitals tend to prefer it over the formula method. In fact, when given the choice between being regulated by budget review or a formula, all New Jersey hospitals chose the former (Worthington 1976). This is indirect evidence that the formula method tends to be tougher on hospitals than the budget method.

Of course, a major difficulty in evaluating impacts of tough versus weak regulatory programs of any sort is that one may expect the tough ones to be implemented in states in which there is political pressure on government to do something about the hospital cost crisis. The precise nature of the regulatory approach may be less important than the political atmosphere existing when the programs are implemented. Unfortunately, there is no way to investigate this empirically.

The extent to which patients in a hospital's market area have insurance covered by revenue-cost controls should bear a direct relationship to the influence of such controls on hospital behavior. This factor is incorporated into our analysis by defining our PR variables as proportions of patients in the market area (such as Medicaid or Blue Cross) covered by particular types of PR; either formula or budget review.

A number of evaluations of state PR programs have been conducted.[11] Among these studies, the most directly relevant empirical results come from Abt Associates and Policy Analysis, Inc. (1976). Holding a number of factors constant, they found that New York PR had no statistically significant impact on wages, using the type of wage measure available from annual AHA surveys. Though insignificant, the PR parameter estimates were uniformly positive, suggesting, if anything, an adverse effect.

To our knowledge, the only other national study of PR is by Sloan and Steinwald (forthcoming, 1980). Overall, the notion that PR is effective in cost containment received no support in that study. If anything, budget-review PR seemed to be more constraining than its formula counterpart, a result that is difficult to rationalize with descriptive evidence on the relative stringency of the two forms of PR regulation.

Utilization Review

In principle, utilization review (UR) serves the dual objective of cost and quality control. In practice, these two objectives conflict.[12] Some measures of quality are cast in terms of utilization (and its associated costs); that is, more quantity is better quality. Hence there is no reason to expect that utilization review systematically reduces hospital costs, especially when the program stresses quality in general, and utilization-oriented indicators of quality in particular. However, it would clearly be unwise to rule out the notion that these programs lower costs *on average* without reference to empirical evidence. The major current federal thrust in this area is the Professional Standards Review Organization (PSRO) program, which was not implemented on a widespread basis until the mid-1970s; thus it is too recent to influence behavior of hospitals in our sample. Our evaluation of UR is confined to reviews undertaken by Blue Cross and state Medicaid agencies.

Data, Empirical Specification, and Estimation

Data

The observational unit for this chapter's empirical analysis is the individual hospital. To be included in the sample, each had to be (1) a nonfederal, short-term general hospital; (2) located within the National Opinion Research

Center's (NORC) Primary Sampling Units (PSU); and (3) a respondent to the AHA's annual survey of hospitals, our core data source, in *each* of seven years, 1969-1975. This selection process yielded a sample of 1,228 hospitals, 21.3 percent of all nonfederal, short-term general hospitals (as of 1975). The use of a cluster rather than a random sample greatly facilitated the task of merging area data from non-AHA sources. Our hospitals come from 34 states (including the District of Columbia) and 250 counties throughout the United States. NORC's PSU framework yields a self-weighting sample of the 1970 U.S. population; our 1,228 hospitals are representative of the consumer population served by nonfederal, short-term general hospitals rather than the hospitals themselves. Compared to all nonfederal, short-term general hospitals, our sample hospitals are larger on average (268 versus 163 beds), more likely to have medical and nursing school affiliations, and less likely to be controlled by local government. Mean occupancy rate and average length of stay are, on average, about 5 to 7 percent higher in sample hospitals. Our analysis encompasses the six-year period, 1970-1975.

Empirical Specification

The dependent variable is the mean annual earnings of hospital employees other than physicians, RNs, LPNs, and trainees, deflated by our area price index. The first set of explanatory variables are hypothesized to affect the demand for the hospital's product and thereby the derived demand for labor in terms of quantity, skill mix, and (at least temporarily) quality-adjusted wages. With one exception, Medicaid, these variables are defined for the hospital's county.[13] The Medicaid variable (MCAID) has been defined for the state, since Medicaid eligibility data are not published at a more disaggregated level. The demand variables are:

INC	Per capita disposable income
DENS	Population per square mile
POPMD	Population per nonfederal, office-based physician
GPPROP	Proportion of these physicians who are general practitioners
POPBD	Population per bed *excluding* beds pertaining to the observational hospital
MCAID	Proportion of population eligible for Medicaid *and* under age 65
MCARE	Proportion of population age 65 and over
INS	Depth of coverage under private health insurance

The first four variables and the Medicaid and Medicare variables have been included in previous studies of hospital behavior and are largely self-explanatory. The INS variable is described in the preceding chapter and in appendix G. The variable POPBD requires elaboration, however.

As beds in other hospitals in the county increase relative to population (POPBD falls), the demand schedule facing our sample hospital should shift inward. Under the standard set of assumptions economists typically propose for firms, this increase should reduce output and, assuming positively sloped cost curves, average costs and inputs should fall. But the standard theory for firms does not suffice. First, the underlying model must take account of salient characteristics of the hospital industry and thereby loses predictive power. Second, much of the competition in the hospital sector is nonprice, and thus costs and input intensity may be *higher* when a hospital faces competitors in its market area. For this reason, POPBD effects in our regressions may well be negative.

Several exogenous (to the hospital) forces on the factor supply side may affect wages. As in previous chapters, we assess the impact of unemployment rates and union activity. The following explanatory variables represent this set of influences:

UN   Unemployment rate in the hospital's PSU

CBREQ   The hospital has received a union request for recognition as a collective bargaining agent.

CBARG   The hospital has a signed collective bargaining agreement covering *any* of its employees.

STR   The hospital has had a strike or other work stoppage.

The unemployment variable takes the value for the SMSA in the case of hospitals in metropolitan PSUs; otherwise, it assumes the value for all areas in the state for which unemployment data are not provided by the BLS. We arrived at the latter estimate by solving an equation with one unknown, the "residual" unemployment rate, and unemployment for selected SMSAs weighted by population and the state's unemployment rate, the knowns. As before, we expect that as UN rises, hospital wages fall; however, as seen in previous chapters, unemployment often has the "wrong" (that is, positive) sign.

As in chapter 4, CBREQ measures the effect of the threat of unionization on hospital costs. STR is a measure of union aggressiveness, which is presumably higher in hospitals that have experienced work stoppages. CBARG, unfortunately, does not measure the extent of unionization in a hospital, only its presence.

Table 5-3 shows the growth in hospital unionization activity during the first half of the 1970s. As is evident from the table, union activity in hospitals grew somewhat over this period, although not dramatically. There are some differences by census division, but there is considerable within-census division variation in table 5-3 as well. The percentages in the table are based on AHA survey data. The method for constructing variables CBARG, CBREQ, and STR from these data is discussed in appendix I.

Hospital characteristics variables include a measure of technical sophistication of the hospital, ASSETB, an asset index, and the following binary variables:

GOVT   Government hospital

PROP   Proprietary hospital

MEDSCH   Medical school-affiliated hospital

NURSCH   Nursing school-affiliated hospital

SIZE1   Bed size < 100

SIZE2 $100 \leqslant$ bed size < 250

SIZE3 $250 \leqslant$ bed size < 400

Hospital characteristic impacts are normalized on voluntary hospitals with 400 beds or more that have neither a medical school nor a nursing school affiliation.

Since plant assets are recorded in terms of original rather than replacement cost, it is necessary to devise a way to hold construction prices constant. Simply deflating by an area price index cannot accomplish this, since assets are accumulated over time. Hence, we developed an asset index by means of an "hedonic" asset regression.

The index was obtained by regressing 1975 net plant assets per bed, deflated by an area price index, on a comprehensive list of binary variables representing hospital facilities and services (for example, cobalt therapy, premature nursery, family planning, home care) and a few other standardizing variables which, with two minor exceptions (beds and beds squared), remain constant from year to year (region, city size, and so on). The estimated parameters from this "hedonic" asset regression indicate the amount of fixed capital associated with specific facilities and services. Since facilities and services vary over time both within and among hospitals, so does ASSETB. This variable should account for a large portion of the variation in skill mix among hospitals. Other hospital characteristics variables, such as ownership, may also pick up skill-mix variations; but as seen in chapter 4, the historical difference between wages paid to government versus private hospital employees (holding occupation constant) has been narrowing over time.

Regulation variables encompass capital-facilities, revenue-cost, and utilization review as well as the proportion of patients in the hospital's market area with cost-based hospital insurance.

Table 5-3
Percent Growth in Hospital Unionization Activity, 1970-1975

	Hospitals with a Signed Collective Bargaining Agreement (CBARG)			Hospitals Receiving a Request for Recognition as a Collective Bargaining Agent during Past Year (CBREQ)			Hospitals Experiencing Job Actions during Past Year (STR)	
	1970	1973	1975	1970	1973	1975	1970	1973
All nonfederal short-term general hospitals	12.3	12.3	14.4	7.7	6.5	17.6	2.0	1.7
New England								
Maine	0.0	0.0	0.0	2.4	0.0	8.2	4.0	0.0
New Hampshire	0.0	0.0	0.0	0.0	0.0	7.4	0.0	0.0
Vermont	0.0	0.0	0.0	0.0	0.0	23.5	0.0	0.0
Massachusetts	22.3	26.5	40.0	17.1	15.6	36.5	2.7	9.1
Rhode Island	0.0	0.0	16.7	0.0	30.0	41.7	0.0	0.0
Connecticut	17.7	20.0	34.3	18.2	11.4	31.4	0.0	0.0
Mid-Atlantic								
New York	40.3	43.0	47.5	19.4	19.8	33.0	6.3	10.1
New Jersey	14.3	13.7	20.6	10.1	15.7	30.4	0.0	5.6
Pennsylvania	1.0	15.7	21.2	8.2	18.1	39.0	2.9	2.5
South Atlantic								
Delaware	0.0	0.0	0.0	16.7	0.0	28.6	0.0	0.0
Maryland	21.43	16.3	17.4	14.6	4.8	13.1	7.1	4.9
District of Columbia	36.4	33.3	36.4	27.3	16.7	36.4	9.1	0.0
Virginia	2.3	3.3	2.2	3.5	3.8	4.4	0.0	0.0
West Virginia	8.1	10.3	8.8	6.5	4.6	25.0	1.6	4.7
North Carolina	0.0	0.8	0.8	0.8	0.0	4.7	2.5	0.0
South Carolina	0.0	0.0	0.0	4.9	0.0	4.3	1.6	0.0
Georgia	0.0	0.0	0.0	1.8	1.6	5.4	0.0	1.6
Florida	0.7	1.2	1.6	2.7	0.6	10.4	3.4	1.3
East North Central								
Ohio	9.8	9.8	13.1	8.7	8.0	30.2	4.0	0.0
Indiana	0.9	0.9	0.9	2.8	0.0	17.1	2.8	1.9
Illinois	10.3	8.8	11.8	8.7	2.8	23.5	3.0	1.9
Michigan	36.2	40.4	44.4	20.0	17.3	25.1	4.0	2.2
Wisconsin	17.4	16.8	17.6	11.4	9.0	11.3	2.8	3.0
East South Central								
Kentucky	6.2	5.8	5.7	1.1	4.3	12.4	3.1	4.3
Tennessee	1.0	1.6	2.4	3.8	1.7	4.8	1.9	3.5
Alabama	1.0	0.0	2.4	1.0	0.0	6.4	1.0	0.9
Mississippi	0.0	0.0	0.0	1.4	0.0	1.0	1.4	0.0
West North Central								
Minnesota	36.8	34.1	40.5	10.8	8.4	12.5	1.8	0.0
Iowa	0.8	0.8	0.8	3.3	0.0	11.2	1.6	0.0
Missouri	8.8	5.8	5.8	5.9	5.5	26.6	2.9	1.8

Table 5-3 *(continued)*

	Hospitals with a Signed Collective Bargaining Agreement (CBARG)			Hospitals Receiving a Request for Recognition as a Collective Bargaining Agent during Past Year (CBREQ)			Hospitals Experiencing Job Actions during Past Year (STR)	
	1970	1973	1975	1970	1973	1975	1970	1973
North Dakota	0.0	0.0	0.0	2.0	0.0	13.5	0.0	0.0
South Dakota	0.0	1.9	1.8	2.0	2.2	3.6	0.0	0.0
Nebraska	0.0	0.0	0.0	2.2	0.0	7.3	0.0	0.0
Kansas	0.0	0.0	2.8	0.8	7.6	2.8	0.8	0.0
West South Central								
Arkansas	1.4	0.0	0.0	1.4	1.2	2.3	0.0	0.0
Louisiana	3.4	2.3	5.3	5.9	2.5	6.8	0.0	0.8
Oklahoma	0.0	0.0	0.0	0.0	0.9	5.1	0.0	0.0
Texas	0.0	0.0	0.0	0.3	0.5	8.3	0.7	0.0
Mountain								
Montana	13.7	11.9	21.1	14.3	3.6	22.8	0.0	0.0
Idaho	0.0	0.0	2.2	2.4	0.0	6.5	0.0	0.0
Wyoming	0.0	0.0	0.0	0.0	0.0	23.1	0.0	0.0
Colorado	3.1	2.7	2.6	3.0	0.0	13.0	0.0	0.0
New Mexico	0.0	0.0	5.6	6.5	2.7	22.2	0.0	0.0
Arizona	5.8	3.5	5.5	3.9	1.8	20.0	0.0	1.8
Utah	0.0	0.0	0.0	0.0	0.0	12.1	0.0	0.0
Nevada	15.4	11.8	23.5	23.1	17.7	29.4	0.0	0.0
Pacific								
Washington	52.0	59.4	64.7	19.2	20.4	40.2	0.0	1.0
Oregon	29.6	33.8	47.3	14.1	17.1	23.0	0.0	0.0
California	25.4	21.5	22.4	12.9	10.4	28.5	1.9	1.6
Alaska	0.0	0.0	6.7	9.1	0.0	20.0	0.0	0.0
Hawaii	45.0	63.2	73.7	25.0	21.1	21.1	25.0	0.0

Source: See appendix I.

Five binary variables represent certificate-of-need (CON) programs. The variable PRECON is one for hospitals located in a state in the year immediately preceding the introduction of CON; thus PRECON can be one for, at most, one of the six years. This variable is designed to account for anticipatory behavior. An operating CON program is classified as either comprehensive or noncomprehensive. As defined, comprehensive programs include service expansion review *and* have a threshold less than $100,000. These programs presumably leave less room for the kind of compensatory impacts reported by Salkever and Bice (1976a, 1976b), such as on growth in assets per bed and/or hospital demand for labor. We make a further distinction between new programs—the first or second year of operation—and mature programs—more than two years of operation. Several states changed from new to mature status during 1970-1975. Thus in a limited way we are able to gauge changes in CON impact as the program matures. It is possible that CON becomes more effective through a form of learning by doing. Prefixes C and N in front of CON designate comprehensive and noncomprehensive programs, respectively; suffixes 1 and 2 identify new and mature programs, respectively.

Most of our remaining regulatory variables operate in conjunction with third-party reimbursement. To construct these variables, a binary variable indicating that the regulatory program exists is multiplied by the proportion of the population in the hospital's area with the kind of insurance to which the regulation in question applies. The variable S1122 is the product of a binary variable indicating whether the program exists in the hospital's state, and the sum of Medicare (MCARE) and Medicaid (MCAID) population proportions (Section 1122 applies to these programs). The variable BCPAA is the product of a binary variable which equals one if the Blue Cross plan in the hospital's area requires local planning agency approval for capital expenditures and Blue Cross' market share in the (Blue Cross plan catchment) area. As previously noted, neither Section 1122 nor the Blue Cross program forbids the hospital from undertaking capital expansion and/or modernization; however, current expenditures associated with these capital purchases can be disallowed.

The ESP program, termed ESP in the analysis and defined as the fraction of the year that ESP was in effect, is the first revenue-cost regulation variable. Formula (FPR) and budget-review (BPR) prospective reimbursement programs are defined as the products of binary variables identifying that the program was in effect and the proportions of the relevant populations covered. Since PR may apply to virtually any type of insurer—and there is substantial interstate variation on this score—we have devoted considerable effort to computing the relevant population proportions.

The variable UR represents hospital utilization review programs developed by Blue Cross and/or Medicaid. It too is weighted by the relevant (Blue Cross and/or Medicaid) population proportions.

Finally, it has often been argued that, on average, cost-based reimbursement is especially inflationary because it gives the hospital a perverse incentive to raise costs.[14] Davis (1973) was rightly critical of past research that simply treated cost-based reimbursement as a binary variable rather than as a proportion representing the population covered by this form of insurance. Yet to date there is no hard evidence that costs are higher where cost-based reimbursement prevails.[15] The variable COSTB is the sum of Medicaid (MCAID) and Medicare (MCARE) population proportions (because these are always cost-based) and the Blue Cross plan area population proportion when the plan uses a cost-based payment method.

To account for unspecified time and regional effects, we include a time trend (TIME), with 1970 equal to 1. Census areas are identified by binary variables NEAST (for northeast), SOUTH, and MIDWEST (North Central). The West is the omitted category.

Functional Form and Estimation

With the exception of the binary hospital characteristics and the regulation variables, which enter linearly, all explanatory variables are in log form. Coefficients associated with variables in logs are elasticities; the remaining coefficients (times one hundred) indicate percentage changes in the dependent variable when the explanatory variable changes from 0 to 1.

Initially, we estimated a dynamic version of the wage relationship, assuming a Koyck lag structure. An implausible negative coefficient on the lagged dependent variable was obtained; the source of the problem appeared to be unusually high values for some of the lagged dependent variable (wage) observations for 1969. Because we do not understand the source of this unanticipated result, we do not present results from the dynamic specification in the next section. Static versions of the equation are presented, however, using a method for pooling time series, cross-section data developed by Nerlove (1971), hereafter termed TSCS. Although the use of a pooling technique is by no means essential for estimating static versions, it has two advantages. First, time-invariant "hospital" or "state" effects are reduced or eliminated. Second, the technique purges the error term of time-dependent serial correlation. This first consideration is potentially important in assessments of the effect of regulation, since regulation may be adopted in areas of persistently high hospital costs and OLS parameters may be positively biased as a result. In the presence of autocorrelated errors, t ratios associated with the estimated coefficients are upward biased.

Empirical Results

Table 5-4 presents four regressions, two estimated by OLS and two by TSCS. Not surprisingly, the OLS regressions have higher R^2s, principally because the estimated parameters pick up hospital-state effects that are omitted in the TSCS regressions. Comparing coefficients from the two sets of regressions, however, the results are reasonably invariant to the technique employed.

As in previous chapters, demand variables play a role in explaining variations in hospital wages. Among the demand variables included, per capita income (INC), population density (DENS), and physician availability (POPMD) have both plausible coefficients and are statistically significant at conventional levels. Density could also be interpreted as a cost-of-living variable; but, as elsewhere in this study, all monetarily expressed variables have been deflated by an area price index, which varies both geographically and temporally.

Neither the private (INS) nor the Medicare (MCARE) insurance variables perform as anticipated. The negative INS and MCARE coefficients persist in all variants we have estimated. It seems best to conclude that during the 1970s,

Table 5-4
Other Employees' Earnings Regressions

Explanatory Variables	OLS (1)	OLS (2)	TSCS (3)	TSCS (4)
INC	0.25* (0.022)	0.14* (0.022)	0.15* (0.032)	0.096* (0.032)
DENS	0.025 (0.019)	0.021* (0.0023)	0.023* (0.0043)	0.019* (0.0045)
POPMD	−0.055* (0.0099)	−0.066* (0.0099)	−0.056* (0.013)	−0.048* (0.013)
GPPROP	0.011 (0.0087)	0.0038 (0.0091)	0.013 (0.174)	−0.022 (0.018)
POPBD	0.0001 (0.0003)	0.0034 (0.0027)	0.0016 (0.017)	0.0015 (0.0048)
MCARE	−0.033* (0.013)	−0.019 (0.014)	−0.042*** (0.027)	−0.030 (0.028)
MCAID	0.0047 (0.0046)	0.018* (0.0057)	0.015** (0.0075)	0.020* (0.0080)
INS	−0.20* (0.013)	−0.11* (0.031)	−0.042** (0.021)	−0.10* (0.025)
ASSETB	0.034* (0.0032)	0.021* (0.0035)	0.0068*** (0.0043)	0.0088** (0.0042)
UN	0.049* (0.0076)	0.078* (0.010)	0.042* (0.0073)	0.10 (0.084)
CBREQ		−0.0088 (0.0064)		−0.0026 (0.0085)
CBARG		0.057* (0.0066)		0.039* (0.019)
STR		0.053* (0.018)		0.098* (0.023)
GOVT		0.011 (0.0074)		
PROP		0.0008 (0.0099)		
MEDSCH		0.059* (0.0062)		
NURSCH		0.045* (0.0069)		
PRECON		0.025* (0.0092)		0.015** (0.0075)
NCON1		0.029* (0.0085)		0.0030 (0.0081)
NCON2		0.028* (0.011)		−0.013 (0.0098)
CCON1		−0.0027 (0.014)		−0.012 (0.013)
CCON2		0.0046 (0.015)		−0.027*** (0.016)

Table 5-4 *(continued)*

Explanatory Variables	OLS (1)	OLS (2)	TSCS (3)	TSCS (4)
S1122		−0.10** (0.042)		−0.12* (0.031)
BCPAA		−0.016 (0.013)		−0.020*** (0.013)
FPR		0.053* (0.018)		0.0022 (0.0034)
BPR		0.015 (0.015)		0.0037 (0.016)
UR		0.062* (0.017)		0.050 (0.042)
COSTB		−0.017 (0.022)		−0.096** (0.040)
ESP		0.063* (0.0062)		0.068* (0.0049)
TIME		−0.0048*** (0.0027)		
NEAST		−0.098* (0.021)		
SOUTH		−0.010 (0.015)		
MIDWEST		0.018 (0.017)		
CONST		8.26	3.59	4.01
	$R^2 = 0.24$ $F(10,5929) = 189.5$	$R^2 = 0.33$ $F(33,5906) = 87.92$	$R^2 = 0.03$ $F(10,5920) = 19.9$	$R^2 = 0.09$ $F(25,5905) = 22.6$

Note: Figures in parentheses are standard errors.

*Significant at the 1 percent level (two-tail test); **Significant at the 5 percent level (two-tail test); ***Significant at the 10 percent level (two-tail test).

insurance in itself has not been responsible for variations in hospital wages (and earnings).

In terms of signs, the union coefficients are fully consistent with the results (using essentially the same specification) reported in chapter 4. As before, the CBREQ coefficients indicate that wages tend to be slightly lower in hospitals receiving requests for collective bargaining coverage. The prospect of unionization in itself ("threat effects") does not appear to be sufficient to raise wages. Both the CBARG and STR parameter estimates are statistically significant at the 1 percent level. The OLS CBARG estimate (variant 2) implies that the presence of a collective bargaining unit raises earnings 6 percent; the corresponding TSCS estimate (variant 4) is about two-thirds of this. By contrast, the TSCS coefficient on STR is higher. Combining the effects of CBARG and STR, coefficients from the second OLS regression imply that an active union (one willing to engage in job actions) boosts earnings 11 percent; from TSCS, the corresponding estimated effect is 14 percent.

The unemployment rate coefficients are uniformly positive. While unanticipated conceptually, we also obtained this result in previous chapters. From all the evidence accumulated in this study, one can safely conclude that adverse conditions in labor markets in the area do not negatively affect hourly wages and annual earnings paid to hospital employees.

The asset index has a positive and significant effect on wages. Although the sign of ASSETB's coefficient was certainly anticipated, we are somewhat surprised that the associated elasticities are negligible. Part of the "technical sophistication effect" may be picked up by MEDSCH and NURSCH in the second OLS regression, but this cannot account for the ASSETB coefficients being small in other regressions as well. The MEDSCH and NURSCH coefficients in the second regression imply that hospitals with medical and nursing school affiliations have average earnings 6 and 5 percent, respectively, above those of hospitals without these affiliations.

In general, the estimated parameters on the regulation variables are lower (more nearly zero if positive, or more negative) using TSCS than OLS, but the differences are not great. Previously, we reported that certificate-of-need programs generally demonstrated no, or even a positive, effect in the Sloan and Steinwald (forthcoming, 1980) study of hospital costs and input use. In this regard, the results on CON in table 5-4 are relatively encouraging. Although the noncomprehensive CON coefficients reveal a now familiar tale, those for comprehensive programs are negative with TSCS as the estimator; and the coefficient on the mature comprehensive CON variable is more negative (CCON2) than its young counterpart (CCON1). The other capital-facilities regulation coefficients are negative and significant in the TSCS regression. In combination, these findings suggest that at least some capital-facilities programs have restrained earnings of hospital employees, presumably through their effect on hospital demand for skilled labor. These results are, on the whole, more favorable to this form of regulation than those reported in our other book (using nonwage dependent variables).

As shown in tables 5-1, 5-2, and in tables in previous chapters, real earnings of hospital employees fell in 1973 and 1974 from their historic highs in 1972. At least in descriptive terms, ESP appears to have been effective during its latter phases. The positive ESP coefficients in table 5-4 serve as a reminder that real earnings were relatively high during part of the ESP period. Because, if anything, ESP regulations had more, rather than fewer, exceptions as the program aged, the rise in real earnings during 1972 must be explained in terms of poor hospital compliance coupled with general effectiveness of ESP in holding down the growth of consumer prices. The positive ESP coefficient is inconsistent with the research by Ginsburg (1976, 1978) discussed earlier in this chapter; but as noted, there are important differences in our empirical approaches.

The parameter estimates on FPR and BPR give no indication that state prospective reimbursement programs have restrained earnings in this sector. In the case of FPR, one could argue that the coefficient represents an omitted New York effect. But the budget-review system was reasonably widespread throughout 1970-1975, and in combination with the use of TSCS, it is difficult to believe that omitted state effects are an important factor. The effect of utilization review (UR) on earnings is positive in both regressions in which UR enters.

Although cost-based reimbursement is often said to be relatively inflationary, the findings on COSTB give no support to this notion. In fact, in the TSCS regression, COSTB's coefficient is both negative and statistically significant at the 5 percent level.

The remaining variables command little policy interest. The TIME parameter estimate suggests that real wages have been declining at the rate of 0.5 percent a year. The Census Area coefficients imply that, in real terms, hospital wages are 8 to 10 percent lower in the Northeast than in other parts of the United States, holding a number of other factors constant. The regional tabulations in table 5-2, of course, did not hold other factors constant.

Summary, Conclusions, and Implications

This chapter has assessed the determinants of mean annual earnings of hospital employees during the 1970s with a special emphasis on the role of regulation and third-party reimbursement. As noted at the outset, the rise in real earnings of hospital employees, on a national basis, has been moderate in recent years; specifically, the growth in real earnings from 1970 through 1975 was 4.9 percent for the entire period, or less than 1 percent per year. This is almost exactly the same as growth in median real family income of male-headed households over the same period (U.S. Department of Commerce 1977). It certainly cannot be said that hospital employees grew rich during these years. As stressed throughout the chapter, one reason for variations in this earnings series is change in skill mix. Yet the trends implied by the AHA data are sufficiently comparable to those derived from other sources for us to conclude that skill-mix changes have not been a *major* influence on average real earnings in the recent past. Breakdowns by census division, presented in table 5-2, indicate some regional variation in both the level and growth in real earnings. In particular, real earnings in the Pacific census division, although the highest, have been declining in relative terms.

In general, past assessments of the impact of various types of regulation on hospital behavior have arrived at rather pessimistic conclusions, at least in terms of cost containment. Not only does regulation seem to be ineffective in achieving its objectives, but there appear to be a number of important unintended and undesirable side effects. But, compared to many previous studies, our results here are less detrimental to hospital regulation. While we find no evidence that state prospective reimbursement programs have depressed real earnings, the results on the Nixon Administration's Economic Stabilization Program (ESP) and capital-facilities regulation are more favorable.

Support for ESP is found in the descriptive evidence rather than in our regressions. After a rise in 1972, real earnings declined. Although there was some catching up in 1975, hospital employees were still worse off in the aggregate in 1975 than in 1972. An alternative specification for ESP, such as Taylor's (1977), which allowed the effectiveness of the program to vary over time, would probably have produced regression results more favorable to ESP. Our descriptive evidence on real earnings is sufficiently convincing for us to concur with Taylor's conclusion that ESP reduced real hospital wages below the levels they would have been in the absence of controls.

Comprehensive certificate-of-need programs that cover many changes in facilities and services, as well as beds, have slightly negative effects on real earnings, presumably through their effects on skill composition. The Section 1122 and Blue Cross Planning Agency approval programs have qualitatively similar effects. Our analysis indicates that both have reduced real hospital earnings, especially Section 1122 programs, in which reductions on the order of 10 to 12 percent emerge from our regression analysis.

There are undoubtedly other important regulatory effects that the AHA data base does not allow one to capture, such as the effect of various types of regulatory controls on wage structure—specifically, relative wages of low- in relation to high-skilled employees. We report on our preliminary evaluation of this issue in the next chapter. But as Schramm (1977) has pointed out, the character of hospital bargaining will undoubtedly continue changing from a bilateral to a multilateral situation with more widespread regulation of hospital costs. State cost-regulating agencies in both New York and Maryland have made their presence felt in collective bargaining.

Our measures of reimbursement fail to show positive effects on earnings. Although the "problem" may be with our insurance measures, another possibility is that insurance had its (inflationary) day during the 1960s. Both the extent and depth of coverage rose rapidly during that decade—and this chapter's analysis only includes observations from the 1970s.

Results on union effects are consistent with findings in earlier chapters, although there are some differences in magnitude of the wage response. To the extent that we can measure them, "threat effects" do not seem to be sources of real wage gains. Once a union is present in the hospital, however, real wages do increase, particularly in combination with strike activity. Hospitals with collective bargaining units are subject to a cost-push force from collective bargaining efforts that policymakers, especially in the regulatory sphere, should take into account.

As in earlier chapters, variables determining demand for the hospital's product have impacts on hospital wages. In this regard, per capita income, population density (though subject to varying interpretations), and physician availability merit particular mention. It appears that demand factors must continue to receive attention as potential sources of labor cost and general inflation in the hospital sector.

Notes

1. General discussions of these issues include Altman and Weiner (1978), Enthoven (1978a, 1978b), Havighurst (1977), and Salkever (1978).

2. Sloan and Steinwald (forthcoming, 1980). This source provides much more detail on variable and file construction than is provided here.

3. Our cost-of-living deflator for converting dollar figures into real terms, equals 1.00 for metropolitan areas of the United States in 1972.

4. See Roemer and Shain (1959), and Roemer (1961).

5. This view is less than fully consistent with a strict constructionist interpretation of "Roemer's law."

6. For details of P.L. 94-641, especially as it applies to CON, see Blumstein and Sloan (1978), and Bovbjerg (1978).

7. U.S. Department of Health, Education, and Welfare (1978).

8. See Kopit et al. (1978).

9. More complete reviews are found in Blumstein and Sloan (1978), and Sloan and Steinwald (forthcoming, 1980).

10. There are several other studies of ESP's effects. See, for example, Altman and Eichenholz (1976), and Furst and Dunkelberg (1978).

11. For a review, see Gaus and Hellinger (1976).

12. For a more detailed review of the cost-quality tradeoff, see Havighurst and Blumstein (1975).

13. Sources of non-AHA variables are given in appendix H.

14. See, for example, Pauly and Drake (1970). Arguments from hospital and insurer perspectives are given by TeKolste (1963), and Sigmond (1963).

15. See Pauly and Drake (1970), Davis (1973), and Salkever (1972). Theoretical discussions of issues related to cost-based reimbursement may be found in Davis (1973), and Sloan and Steinwald (forthcoming, 1980).

6

Occupation-Specific Wage Trends in Large Hospitals: An Analysis of Vanderbilt University's Surveys of Hospital Wages

Background

There is a regrettable lack of detailed data on hospital wages at the level of the hospital and/or small community. Researchers and policymakers in need of such data have been forced to use the American Hospital Association's annual surveys—our data base for the analysis in Chapter 5. Although AHA data have the dual advantages of being current and available at a low level of aggregation, they also have the important deficiency that wages for specific occupations or skill levels are not reported. Therefore variations in hospitals' payroll expenditures per full-time equivalent employee cannot be linked to changes in occupation and skill mix.

For certain purposes, this shortcoming may not be serious. If the objective of public policy is to curtail the growth of hospital costs in general and hospital labor costs in particular, there may be comparatively little concern about the degree to which mean wage changes reflect changes in employee composition versus movements in pure wages. But in other contexts, the AHA data may be too crude. Some changes in mean wages are surely due to technological innovations and to changes in hospital production functions. Sophisticated new equipment requires skilled employees for operation and maintenance. Increased sharing of services among hospitals and purchase of services on a contract basis (such as laundry and housekeeping) bring about changes in employee mix. Such changes will affect mean wages, but will have no bearing on wages adjusted for occupation and skill mix.

More specific concerns relate to the consequences of particular regulatory programs and market developments. For example, under a state prospective reimbursement program or nationally imposed wage and price controls, it would be desirable to ascertain the types of employees that would be affected by various exemptions. As noted in chapter 5, low-wage workers were exempted from Economic Stabilization Program controls. Moreover, one may want to assess the effect of previous exemptions. For instance, under ESP did wages of low-skilled workers rise in relative terms? In gauging the effects of collective bargaining, it is useful to link specific wages with occupations covered. The BLS data analyzed in chapter 3 allowed us to do this, and we saw that the strength of the wage response to unions varied from occupation to occupation. Other examples could be mentioned, but we strongly suspect that most readers already agree that it is desirable to have occupation-specific wage data.

The Vanderbilt University (VU) Personnel Department has conducted hospital wage surveys annually from 1970 to the present, with the exception of 1975. These national surveys have been limited to nonfederal, short-term general hospitals with four hundred beds or more. Minimum and maximum wage data are routinely collected for about seventy occupations; the exact number varies slightly from year to year. Wage data pertain to health sector-specific occupations, such as RNs, LPNs, and medical technicians, as well as the more general categories of secretaries, clerks, and cleaners. For most types of workers, wages are recorded by skill level (for example, Clerk-Typist I, Clerk-Typist II, Clerk-Typist III). Job definitions have been included with the mail questionnaire in all years, thus reducing possible ambiguity in job titles.

This chapter provides an assessment of the VU data. To the extent comparisons with other data bases are possible, results from the VU data are basically consistent with those from our other sources. Perhaps most striking, and counter to conventional wisdom, is that real occupation-specific starting and maximum wages paid hospital employees have declined in the 1970s. In other words, holding occupation and job tenure constant, the financial position of hospital workers appears to have deteriorated in terms of keeping up with inflation. Limitations and qualifications pertaining to this finding are discussed in this chapter.

In the following section we describe the VU data base in greater detail. The next section presents descriptive evidence on money (nominal) and real wages in specific occupations over the 1970-1977 period, followed by a simple analysis of associations between union presence and wages. In the final section we summarize our findings and briefly indicate how the VU data (or similar data) could be used in future research.

The Vanderbilt University Data Base

At the outset, it must be recognized that, although they provide unique, occupation-specific wage information, the VU surveys were neither conceived nor conducted for the purpose of scholarly research. Rather, the primary purpose of the VU surveys has been to provide information to the university for guidance in establishing its own wage-setting policies. While the surveys provide valuable data, we have also had to deal with some imperfections in the VU data base arising from lack of adherence to survey research principles. These imperfections are not devastating; but they do require us to take some steps to ensure that estimates derived from the surveys are meaningful, as well as care in interpretation.

All surveys have been initiated in the fall of each year, with varying degrees of follow-up. The personnel department attempted to survey all U.S. short-term general hospitals with four hundred beds or more, but it is likely that not all such hospitals were sent questionnaires in some years. We are not certain how many questionnaires were sent, but we do know that the response rates were rather low, particularly in the years 1971 through 1974. Table 6-1 provides information on usable responses in each year by census division, plus the distribution of the sampling universe (that is, all short-term, nonfederal hospitals with four hundred beds or more) by census division as of 1976. The latter column is provided to indicate the proportions of the universe sampled by census division.

It is immediately apparent from table 6-1 that the number of responses to VU surveys across years is extremely variable. We do not know what the actual response rates were because mailing lists for earlier surveys have not been kept, but it is clear that the proportions of sample-eligible hospitals from which usable responses were obtained is also extremely variable across census divisions. This is indicated by our 1976 data. What is not explicitly shown, but is apparent from examination of the table entries, is that the percentages sampled by census division change markedly from year to year. It is therefore obviously incorrect to use these data in raw form to compute intertemporal changes in wage scales. To do so would introduce substantial error in the time series due to pure wage variations across census divisions.

To deal with the problem of unequal distribution of responses by census division over time, we have adjusted all of the wage data into East South Central (ESC) equivalents. Intuitively, this means that a minimum or maximum wage paid to employees in a specific job category in a census division other than East

Table 6-1

Number of Usable Responses to VU Surveys by Census Division and Year, 1970-1977; Sampling Universe and Percent of Universe Sampled by Census Division, 1976

	1970	1971	1972	1973	1974	1976	1977	Sampling Universe 1976	Percent of Universe Sampled 1976
New England	10	5	8	5	0	6	7	24	25.0
Mid-Atlantic	20	6	5	14	0	32	38	117	27.4
South Atlantic	38	22	21	30	21	33	41	89	37.1
East North Central	40	24	23	26	21	54	58	134	40.3
East South Central	11	9	8	17	8	27	26	33	81.8
West North Central	23	14	15	14	11	25	28	51	49.0
West South Central	18	8	5	12	8	18	15	41	43.9
Mountain	8	4	4	5	0	9	7	13	69.2
Pacific	14	3	3	2	0	11	13	38	28.9
All	182	95	92	125	69	215	233	540	39.8

South Central is altered in proportion to the "pure" real wage differential existing between ESC and the other census division. Estimates of region-specific pure real wage differentials are taken from the 1970 census regressions pertaining to hospital industry employees presented in chapter 4, table 4-5 (regressions one and five). The regressions hold constant a wide range of factors related to employee quality (education, experience, and so on); the coefficients of the census division dummy variables in these regressions represent region-specific wage differentials not accounted for by the other explanatory variables. Our conversion of wages into ESC dollars is based entirely on the census division coefficients from the two table 4-5 regressions. For male hospital employees, this adjustment most often meant *raising* real wages of hospital employees in other census divisions to arrive at the ESC real wage; in the case of females, 1970 ESC real wages were, other things being equal, fairly much in the middle of the national wage distribution. Thus the conversion involved raising real wages in some census divisions and lowering them in others. The proportion of males and females in each occupation listed in the VU surveys was estimated and used as weights in applying the census division adjustment coefficients to the VU wage data.

The advantages of adjusting the VU wage data in this manner outweigh its limitations, but some of the limitations merit brief mention. First, the census regressions are based on data pertaining to the broad category, hospital employees, without regard to specific occupations; region-specific real wage differentials may vary among census divisions. Second, the male/female proportion estimates used in the adjustments are necessarily somewhat crude. Third, the within-census division geographic distributions of employees are assumed to be the same for census and VU survey data. Fourth, the pure wage differentials estimated for 1970 are assumed to hold for all years, 1970 through 1977. Fifth, the means are expressed in terms of ESC dollars rather than in national mean minimum and maximum wages for specific occupations. Nonetheless, the primary research value of these data is to compare money (undeflated) and real (deflated) wages and trace wage movements over time, and this could not be done reliably without adjustment of the raw wage data. The following two sections present evidence on occupation-specific wages based on East South Central equivalent wage data from the VU surveys.

Descriptive Evidence on Hospital Employees' Wages

In this section we present and discuss selected wage data from the VU surveys. Our discussion centers on table 6-2 which contains money and real minimum and maximum wage averages for eighteen hospital occupations. Not all of the seventy or so occupations are presented to avoid information overload. We selected the occupations shown in table 6-2 on the basis of the following criteria:

1. Data were available for each of the seven years.
2. The occupations selected are frequently reported; that is, relatively few hospitals failed to report these wages.
3. Occupations selected are relatively "important" in terms of number of persons employed.
4. A wide range of wages, from relatively low-paid to relatively high-paid employees, are represented.
5. Occupations selected are representative of a broad range of employee types, including nursing, other professional and technical, clerical, and low-skilled employees.

For each occupation, table 6-2 gives money and real minimum and maximum ESC equivalent wages. Real wages are money wages deflated by an area price index.[1] The index corrects for both geographic and intertemporal variations in price levels; it was constructed such that the index mean for sample hospitals in 1972 is 1.00. Deflating (division) by the index raises pre-1972 figures and lowers post-1972 figures, enabling us to determine, in any year, to what extent wage scale increases have kept up with general inflation in the economy.

Principal Findings

From table 6-2 it is apparent that wage scale increases have not kept up with general price level increases; nearly all of the changes in minimum and maximum real wages from around 1972 on are negative, a result consistent with all time series evidence on hospital wages presented in previous chapters. Here we list our principal findings from examination of the table:

1. The money wage scale increased consistently over the period, with a tendency toward a slowdown in 1973-1974, the latter ESP period. With a few exceptions, the increases between 1970 and 1977 were between 40 and 55 percent.

2. The real wage scale, with only two exceptions in the 18 occupations listed, *decreased* over the 1970-1977 period. In nearly every instance, the peak real wage, for both minimum and maximum cases, occurred in 1972 or 1973.

3. The range between minimum and maximum wages tended to broaden over the 1970-1977 period. In nearly every case, the increase in money wage was greater for maximum than for minimum wages, and the decrease in real wage was less for maximum than minimum wages.

4. There is very little evidence of systematic differences in wage trends by

Table 6-2
Trends in Money and Real Minimum and Maximum Wages for Selected Hospital Occupations, 1970-1977

	Custodian				Clerk I			
	Minimum		Maximum		Minimum		Maximum	
	Money	Real	Money	Real	Money	Real	Money	Real
1970	2.27	2.44	2.75	2.95	2.36	2.52	2.90	3.10
1971	2.36	2.45	2.87	2.99	2.46	2.54	3.04	3.15
1972	2.51	2.51	3.05	3.05	2.56	2.56	3.16	3.16
1973	2.63	2.48	3.28	3.07	2.66	2.51	3.35	3.16
1974	2.64	2.32	3.25	2.86	2.78	2.41	3.53	3.05
1976	3.18	2.35	3.88	2.87	3.32	2.44	4.13	3.02
1977	3.36	2.31	4.13	2.84	3.49	2.40	4.36	2.99
Percent Change 1970-1977	48.0	−5.3	50.1	−3.7	47.9	−4.8	50.3	−3.5

	Nurse Aide				EKG Technician			
	Minimum		Maximum		Minimum		Maximum	
	Money	Real	Money	Real	Money	Real	Money	Real
1970	2.45	2.62	3.00	3.22	2.67	2.87	3.23	3.58
1971	2.57	2.67	3.21	3.34	2.72	2.82	3.44	3.57
1972	2.71	2.71	3.36	3.36	2.93	2.93	3.72	3.72
1973	2.89	2.72	3.65	3.42	3.07	2.89	3.90	3.67
1974	2.88	2.57	3.60	3.21	3.01	2.66	3.84	3.40
1976	3.50	2.57	4.32	3.18	3.67	2.70	4.58	3.37
1977	3.72	2.55	4.62	3.17	3.96	2.71	4.93	3.38
Percent Change 1970-1977	51.8	−2.7	54.0	−1.6	48.3	−5.6	52.6	−5.6

	Security Officer				LPN			
	Minimum		Maximum		Minimum		Maximum	
	Money	Real	Money	Real	Money	Real	Money	Real
1970	2.95	3.16	3.58	3.85	3.09	3.31	3.83	4.10
1971	3.07	3.20	3.87	4.05	3.20	3.32	4.08	4.22
1972	3.29	3.29	4.09	4.09	3.41	3.41	4.29	4.29
1973	3.38	3.19	4.21	3.96	3.53	3.33	4.50	4.22
1974	3.33	2.97	4.27	3.81	3.59	3.20	4.57	4.07
1976	3.96	2.90	4.94	3.64	4.27	3.14	5.35	3.93
1977	4.18	2.86	5.31	3.64	4.51	3.10	5.69	3.91
Percent Change 1970-1977	41.7	−9.5	48.3	−5.5	46.0	−6.3	48.6	−4.6

Table 6-2 *(continued)*

| | Secretary II | | | | Respiratory Therapist | | | |
| | Minimum | | Maximum | | Minimum | | Maximum | |
	Money	Real	Money	Real	Money	Real	Money	Real
1970	3.11	3.34	3.91	4.21	3.17	3.40	3.95	4.24
1971	3.24	3.35	4.10	4.24	3.23	3.35	4.17	4.32
1972	3.44	3.44	4.33	4.33	3.53	3.53	4.43	4.43
1973	3.57	3.36	4.58	4.31	3.78	3.52	4.83	4.48
1974	3.63	3.18	4.63	4.07	3.85	3.33	4.90	4.25
1976	4.35	3.18	5.51	4.04	4.48	3.29	5.62	4.13
1977	4.59	3.15	5.82	3.99	5.29	3.62	6.77	4.64
Percent Change								
1970-1977	47.6	−5.7	48.9	−5.2	66.9	6.5	71.4	9.4

| | Social Worker I | | | | Medical Technician II | | | |
| | Minimum | | Maximum | | Minimum | | Maximum | |
	Money	Real	Money	Real	Money	Real	Money	Real
1970	4.65	4.10	4.85	5.16	4.07	4.34	5.10	5.46
1971	3.84	4.14	5.08	5.24	4.19	4.34	5.31	5.50
1972	4.23	4.23	5.40	5.40	4.38	4.38	5.53	5.53
1973	4.37	4.07	5.54	5.14	4.66	4.35	5.96	5.55
1974	4.48	3.81	5.81	4.92	4.89	4.15	6.26	5.32
1976	5.08	3.74	6.57	4.83	5.44	3.99	6.97	5.13
1977	5.36	3.69	6.91	4.75	5.73	3.93	7.35	5.06
Percent Change								
1970-1977	15.3	−10.0	42.5	−7.9	40.8	−9.4	44.1	−7.3

| | Accountant I | | | | RN | | | |
| | Minimum | | Maximum | | Minimum | | Maximum | |
	Money	Real	Money	Real	Money	Real	Money	Real
1970	4.02	4.33	5.07	5.46	4.24	4.55	5.25	5.61
1971	4.27	4.42	5.41	5.60	4.36	4.54	5.52	5.73
1972	4.49	4.49	5.74	5.74	4.56	4.56	5.74	5.74
1973	4.63	4.35	5.99	5.58	4.85	4.53	6.18	5.75
1974	4.71	4.21	6.06	5.42	4.97	4.35	6.34	5.55
1976	5.52	4.04	7.22	5.28	5.72	4.21	7.25	5.33
1977	5.76	3.94	7.53	5.17	6.04	4.15	7.69	5.28
Percent Change								
1970-1977	43.3	−9.0	48.5	−5.3	42.5	−9.5	46.5	−5.9

Table 6-2 *(continued)*

| | Physical Therapist | | | | Programmer II | | | |
| | Minimum | | Maximum | | Minimum | | Maximum | |
	Money	Real	Money	Real	Money	Real	Money	Real
1970	4.47	4.80	5.61	6.00	4.55	4.90	5.87	6.29
1971	4.60	4.77	5.85	6.06	4.66	4.84	6.08	6.26
1972	4.89	4.89	6.18	6.18	4.94	4.94	6.30	6.30
1973	5.11	4.77	6.53	6.05	5.33	5.01	6.95	6.45
1974	5.35	4.67	6.93	6.04	5.05	4.56	6.52	5.84
1976	6.08	4.47	7.76	5.71	6.15	4.53	8.00	5.84
1977	6.39	4.39	8.23	5.66	6.51	4.47	8.52	5.81
Percent Change 1970-1977	43.0	−8.5	46.7	−5.7	43.0	−8.8	45.1	−7.7

| | Dietitian | | | | Head Nurse | | | |
| | Minimum | | Maximum | | Minimum | | Maximum | |
	Money	Real	Money	Real	Money	Real	Money	Real
1970	4.51	4.82	5.73	6.11	4.90	5.25	6.03	6.45
1971	4.66	4.83	5.95	6.14	5.02	5.21	6.30	6.52
1972	4.95	4.95	6.24	6.24	5.28	5.28	6.66	6.66
1973	5.18	4.82	6.71	6.22	5.63	5.25	7.21	6.71
1974	5.45	4.72	7.07	6.11	5.72	5.04	7.34	6.45
1976	6.04	4.43	7.76	5.68	6.60	4.85	8.47	6.22
1977	6.38	4.37	8.26	5.65	7.03	4.83	9.07	6.23
Percent Change 1970-1977	41.5	−9.3	44.2	−7.5	43.5	−8.0	50.4	−3.4

| | Nurse Anesthetist | | | | Pharmacist | | | |
| | Minimum | | Maximum | | Minimum | | Maximum | |
	Money	Real	Money	Real	Money	Real	Money	Real
1970	5.47	5.88	6.77	7.24	5.53	5.93	6.72	7.19
1971	5.72	5.96	7.31	7.60	5.68	5.89	7.06	7.33
1972	6.05	6.05	7.69	7.69	6.08	6.08	7.54	7.54
1973	6.66	6.24	8.60	7.95	6.54	6.11	8.32	7.69
1974	7.11	6.22	8.91	7.76	6.58	5.82	8.51	7.36
1976	8.02	5.87	10.10	7.32	7.63	5.64	9.64	7.06
1977	8.63	5.98	11.11	7.57	8.02	5.50	10.18	6.97
Percent Change 1970-1977	57.8	1.7	64.1	4.6	45.0	−7.3	51.5	−3.1

type of occupation. Nursing occupations appear to have experienced less of a decline in real minimum wages than other technical-professional occupations, clerical less than nontechnical, nonclerical occupations, and female-dominated less than male-dominated occupations; however, these differences are relatively slight and well within normal ranges of statistical tolerance.

5. There is some evidence of differential wage experience by wage level. For example, by dividing the eighteen occupations into two groups corresponding to the lowest and highest minimum wages in 1972, we find that the real minimum wage average decrease from 1970 to 1977 was 4.8 percent for the low-wage group, while the corresponding figure was 7.6 percent for the high-wage group. This tendency is investigated in depth later.[2]

Relative Real Wage Performance

The issue of relative performance of real wages in high- and low-paid hospital occupations clearly has policy relevance. For example, low-paid hospital employees were exempted from control under the Economic Stabilization Program (ESP) of the early 1970s. Further, recently proposed wage-price guidelines by the Carter Administration exempt low-wage workers. Policymakers have made it clear that they do not wish controls placed on hospital cost increases to impose financial hardships on low-income workers, of which hospitals are a significant employer. Thus particularly in the face of declining real wages, the relative performance of low-wage hospital occupations should be of interest to those concerned with hospital cost inflation.

To further investigate this issue, we identified fifty-three occupations for which data were available from the VU surveys in all survey years. For these occupations we have computed Pearson product-moment and Spearman rank-order correlation coefficients between the 1972 minimum real wage level and the corresponding real wage change between 1970 and 1977. The product-moment coefficient is -0.26, statistically significant at slightly less than the 5 percent level. The rank-order coefficient is $-.56$, statistically significant at the 1 percent level. The difference between the two correlations is probably due to the presence of a few extreme values which affect the product-moment coefficient substantially more than the rank-order one. The correlation analysis implies that there is a definite negative association between wage scale levels and rates of change, and that over the 1970-1977 period low-wage occupations fared relatively better than their high-wage counterparts.[3]

One cannot tell, based on VU data, what has happened to mean wages of individual hospital employees over the 1970-1977 period. Because these data define occupation-specific wage ranges, they do not indicate the average wage within the range. Yet, as discussed in greater detail in chapter 7, the trends displayed in table 6-2 are quite consistent with those presented in previous chapters. Over time, individual employees may obtain wage increases greater than the wage range increase by moving up within the range. Employees may also realize real wage increases by changing occupations; particularly given that most of the occupations have multiple grades (for example, Clerks I through IV, Lab Technicians I and II). Based on data presented in previous chapters, however, it appears that the realization of such opportunities has not out-weighed the overall decline in real wage scales. On the whole, the VU surveys are consistent with, and add to, prior evidence of a decline in real hospital wages during much of the 1970s.

Unionization and Hospital Wages

Having examined real wage scale changes over the 1970 to 1977 period for specific hospital occupations, a logical next step is to identify factors that exert an influence over these trends. The availability of some hospital-specific unionization data from the AHA and VU surveys provides a means of investigating associations between wage changes and union coverage in hospitals.

In earlier chapters and elsewhere (Sloan and Steinwald, forthcoming 1980), using several alternative data sources, we have established that unions exert a positive influence on hospital wages as well as on labor and total costs. In this section we further describe the influence of unions on occupation-specific wage scales. Because hospital employees are heterogeneous in terms of job types, skill levels, and so on, several unions might be represented in a single hospital; and hospitals with unions may vary considerably in types and percentages of employees covered. Thus, identifying individual hospitals as unionized or nonunionized is only a rough approximation—a more complete examination of union influence requires a look at occupation-specific union activity.

The 1973 AHA "*Special Topics*" survey obtained information from hospi-tals on types of employees covered by unions, including maintenance, house-keeping, dietary, RN nursing, non-RN nursing, and some catch-all categories such as "all nonsupervisory/professional." Individual hospital responses to this survey were merged with the VU wage data.[4] Similar unionization information was collected from VU survey respondents in 1976 and 1977 via supplemental questionnaires. Thus, for some occupations, we are able to examine relationships between unionization status and wages in three years—1973, 1976, and 1977. For all VU survey respondents in 1976 and 1977, we are able to determine if these occupations were unionized in 1973. Our data do not permit us to follow the wage experience of a cohort of hospitals over time because few hospitals have responded to each of the surveys. Our comparisons contain hospitals in the later years not included in the earlier years and vice versa; the criterion for inclusion is that we have the requisite collective bargaining and wage informa-tion. The data do permit cross-sectional comparisons and provide some indica-tions of relationships between intertemporal wage scale changes and union-ization.

Table 6-3 presents wage scale data for three employee groups: house-keeping, non-RN nursing, and RN nursing. To enhance intertemporal compar-ability of wage scales between unionized and nonunionized hospitals, we report only real East South Central equivalent minimum and maximum wages. The table presents wage scale means pertaining to nonunionized and unionized occupations in 1973 and 1977. The 1977 unionized occupation wage means are divided into those that pertain to nonunionized and unionized occupations in 1973. This enables us to compare the once-and-for-all impact of unions on wage scales with their long-term effect. Numbers of cases are shown to give an indication of the relative importance of unionization in different occupations; these numbers may also have meaning to some readers concerned with statistical confidence.[5] The percent change figures pertain to employee groups that were nonunionized in both 1973 and 1977, and those that were unionized in both 1973 and 1977. Our chief findings from examination of table 6-3 are the following:

1. In our sample of 400+ bed hospitals, the mean proportion of hospitals whose housekeeping and non-RN nursing employees were unionized was between 18 and 19 percent in 1973, and grew a modest amount, generally less than 1 percent per year, between 1973 and 1977. In contrast, the mean proportion of hospitals whose RN nursing employees were unionized was generally less than 10 percent in 1973, but more than doubled over the 1973 to 1977 period.

2. Mean ESC-equivalent wages consistently tend to be higher for unionized than for nonunionized employees, sometimes over 20 percent higher. This tendency is strongest for lower skill occupation minimum wages in 1973 and weakest for RN nursing occupation maximum wages in 1977.

3. Mean minimum and maximum real wages tend to decrease *less* overtime for nonunionized than for unionized employees. The difference in real wage decreases tends to be greatest for mean minimum wages of lower skill occupations.

4. One curious result in table 6-3 pertains to the mean 1977 wage scales of hospitals with occupations either unionized or nonunionized in 1973. We find evidence of a once-and-for-all positive effect of unions on wage scales in that wages paid to unionized occupations that were not unionized in 1973 tend to be above wages paid to occupations not unionized throughout the period. However, the once-and-for-all effect is not the only effect because wages paid to occupations unionized throughout the period tend to be higher than those paid to occupations that became unionized during the period. This is curious in light of the fact that the wage differential between unionized and nonunionized employees tends to narrow over time. Several factors might account for this phenomenon, but we cannot identify these with existing data; this will have to await more thorough research in the future.[6]

Summary and Implications

In this chapter we have presented previously unreported descriptive evidence on occupation-specific wage scales in large hospitals over the 1970 to 1977 period.

Table 6-3
East South Central Equivalent Real Wage Scales and Wage Scale Changes, 1973 to 1977, for Selected Hospital Occupations, by Unionization Status[a]

Union Group I: Housekeeping

Custodian

	Minimum ESC Equivalent Wage						Maximum ESC Equivalent Wage					
	Nonunion		Union (1977)				Nonunion		Union (1977)			
			Nonunion (1973)		Union (1973)				Nonunion (1973)		Union (1973)	
	Wage	(n)	Wage	(n)	Wage	(n)	Wage	(n)	Wage	(n)	Wage	(n)
1973	2.39	(96)	2.44	(19)	2.89	(22)	3.01	(87)	2.80	(17)	3.35	(20)
1977	2.25	(177)			2.58	(32)	2.80	(172)			3.05	(29)
Percent Change	−5.9				−10.7		−7.0				−9.0	

Maid

	Minimum ESC Equivalent Wage						Maximum ESC Equivalent Wage					
	Nonunion		Union (1976)				Nonunion		Union (1976)			
			Nonunion (1973)		Union (1973)				Nonunion (1973)		Union (1973)	
	Wage	(n)	Wage	(n)	Wage	(n)	Wage	(n)	Wage	(n)	Wage	(n)
1973	2.52	(93)	2.56	(13)	3.09	(21)	3.18	(85)	2.98	(13)	3.59	(19)
1976[b]	2.44	(165)			2.70	(22)	3.01	(158)			3.16	(20)
Percent Change	−3.2				−12.6		−5.3				−12.0	

Union Group II: Non-RN Nursing

Nurse-Aide

Minimum ESC Equivalent Wage

| | Nonunion | | Union (1977) | | | |
| | | | Nonunion (1973) | | Union (1973) | |
	Wage	(n)	Wage	(n)	Wage	(n)
1973	2.61	(97)			3.18	(22)
1977	2.50	(177)	2.71	(20)	2.72	(27)
Percent Change	−4.2				−14.5	

Maximum ESC Equivalent Wage

| | Nonunion | | Union (1977) | | | |
| | | | Nonunion (1973) | | Union (1973) | |
	Wage	(n)	Wage	(n)	Wage	(n)
1973	3.33	(89)			3.78	(20)
1977	3.16	(173)	3.21	(18)	3.21	(24)
Percent Change	−5.1				−15.1	

LPN

Minimum ESC Equivalent Wage

| | Nonunion | | Union (1977) | | | |
| | | | Nonunion (1973) | | Union (1973) | |
	Wage	(n)	Wage	(n)	Wage	(n)
1973	3.25	(100)			3.69	(22)
1977	3.06	(183)	3.12	(20)	3.32	(30)
Percent Change	−5.8				−10.0	

Maximum ESC Equivalent Wage

| | Nonunion | | Union (1977) | | | |
| | | | Nonunion (1973) | | Union (1973) | |
	Wage	(n)	Wage	(n)	Wage	(n)
1973	4.14	(92)			4.55	(21)
1977	3.91	(179)	3.83	(18)	3.96	(28)
Percent Change	−5.6				−13.0	

Table 6-3 *(continued)*

Union Group III: RN Nursing

RN

Minimum ESC Equivalent Wage

| | Nonunion | | Union (1977) | | | |
| | | | Nonunion (1973) | | Union (1973) | |
	Wage	(n)	Wage	(n)	Wage	(n)
1973	4.50	(111)			4.93	(10)
1977	4.13	(190)	4.23	(18)	4.35	(22)
Percent Change	−8.2				−11.8	

Maximum ESC Equivalent Wage

| | Nonunion | | Union (1977) | | | |
| | | | Nonunion (1973) | | Union (1973) | |
	Wage	(n)	Wage	(n)	Wage	(n)
1973	5.72	(103)			5.98	(9)
1977	5.29	(187)	5.19	(16)	5.29	(22)
Percent Change	−7.5				−11.5	

Assistant Head Nurse

Minimum ESC Equivalent Wage

| | Nonunion | | Union (1977) | | | |
| | | | Nonunion (1973) | | Union (1973) | |
	Wage	(n)	Wage	(n)	Wage	(n)
1973	4.90	(70)			5.41	(9)
1977	4.53	(106)	4.69	(12)	4.88	(18)
Percent Change	−7.6				−9.8	

Maximum ESC Equivalent Wage

| | Nonunion | | Union (1977) | | | |
| | | | Nonunion (1973) | | Union (1973) | |
	Wage	(n)	Wage	(n)	Wage	(n)
1973	6.26	(67)			6.43	(8)
1977	5.79	(104)	5.72	(12)	5.95	(17)
Percent Change	−7.5				−7.5	

Head Nurse

Minimum ESC Equivalent Wage

	Nonunion		Union (1977)			
			Nonunion (1973)		Union (1973)	
	Wage	(n)	Wage	(n)	Wage	(n)
1973	5.22	(110)			5.64	(9)
1977	4.81	(174)	4.87	(18)	5.00	(21)
Percent Change	−7.9				−11.3	

Maximum ESC Equivalent Wage

	Nonunion		Union (1977)			
			Nonunion (1973)		Union (1973)	
	Wage	(n)	Wage	(n)	Wage	(n)
1973	6.71	(103)			6.69	(8)
1977	6.27	(170)	6.16	(17)	6.05	(20)
Percent Change	−6.6				−9.6	

Nursing Supervisor

Minimum ESC Equivalent Wage

	Nonunion		Union (1977)			
			Nonunion (1973)		Union (1973)	
	Wage	(n)	Wage	(n)	Wage	(n)
1973	5.65	(100)			6.19	(8)
1977	5.21	(168)	5.24	(17)	5.46	(17)
Percent Change	−7.8				−11.8	

Maximum ESC Equivalent Wage

	Nonunion		Union (1977)			
			Nonunion (1973)		Union (1973)	
	Wage	(n)	Wage	(n)	Wage	(n)
1973	7.41	(90)			7.39	(7)
1977	6.84	(162)	6.70	(16)	7.02	(17)
Percent Change	−7.7				−5.0	

Data Sources: VU Surveys, 1973, 1976, and 1977; AHA Special Topics Survey, 1973.

aData pertain only to four-hundred-plus bed hospitals.

b1977 data not available.

Our chief finding is that real wage scales reached their peak in 1972-1973, but generally declined over the entire period. This was true of both minimum and maximum wages, but especially the former. We also presented evidence that low-paid workers have fared better than highly paid ones over the period—a finding that is likely to provide some encouragement to policymakers who have wished to avoid imposing financial hardships on low-income workers via the various hospital cost containment strategies implemented during the years studied.

The VU data also provide strong support for other evidence that unions exert a positive influence on hospital wage scales, suggesting there will be increasing inflationary pressure in the future as unions become more prevalent in hospitals. This prospect is mitigated somewhat by the concurrent finding that union/nonunion wage scale differences tend to diminish over time. Moreover, that such differences tend to be greatest for low-income workers is also likely to make this prospect more palatable to policymakers.

The availability of occupation-specific wage data at a low level of aggregation provides several opportunities for research in hospital economics. On one hand, while we have used these data only descriptively in the present study, such data might be employed in more detailed analyses of hospital labor markets. One would want to know what factors, other than unions, influence wage trends; for example, extending chapter 5's analysis further, does regulation of hospitals, including prospective reimbursement and certificate-of-need programs, influence hospital wage scales? If so, which types of occupation are influenced the most? It is possible that regulatory programs, along with the ESP, are, in part, responsible for wage scale trends exhibited in table 6-2.

In addition, occupation-specific wage data are extremely useful in more general analyses of hospital costs and input choices. Prevailing wage scales, for example, may influence hospitals to change from direct provision of certain services to a contract or shared basis for these services. Wage scales may also affect input intensity and, ultimately, the nature of the hospital product.

Thus while the VU data are imperfect from a survey research standpoint, they represent a definite step in the right direction. There clearly exists a need to understand factors underlying the inflationary trend in hospital costs; and a complete data base on labor input prices, available at the individual hospital level and over time, is a necessary ingredient for furthering this understanding.

Notes

1. The index is described in appendix A.

2. Even though these differences in percentages appear substantial, it is risky to conclude anything on the basis of these figures alone. If the occupations are grouped into thirds by minimum wage in 1972, and the average real wage

decreases of the upper and lower third compared, the differences in percentage decreases in real wages are *less* than those of the two-group comparison. In this case, it is clearly sensible to take advantage of the whole of the data available to us rather than rely on the "selected occupations" data.

3. We have considered but rejected the notion that this interpretation is subject to regression fallacy. Nevertheless, due to the fact that the average minimum wage levels are unweighted means (that is, all occupations are given the same weight) and to the other data limitations mentioned, this interpretation should not be accepted uncritically.

4. Because the AHA attempts to survey all U.S. hospitals, we were able to match nearly all of our VU survey respondents with corresponding information from the AHA survey.

5. Because the VU sample is nonrandom, we thought it inappropriate to perform means tests on wage estimates in table 6-3. In general, the differences that we discuss in the text are sufficiently great that there is very little risk of ascribing substantive meaning to chance results.

6. One explanation would suggest different effects of unions in relation to the year of unionization; that is, hospitals and occupations unionized relatively recently experience different wage trends than those unionized in the past. Another type of explanation depends on nonlinearities in relative wage experiences of unionized and nonunionized occupations over time; for example, union wages may perform relatively well for a period immediately following unionization and then relatively poorly (particularly if there is a catch-up phenomenon affecting nonunion wages) thereafter.

7

Summary and Implications

It seldom happens in empirical research that one has the opportunity or resources to use several independent sources of data to investigate a complex issue such as wage setting in hospitals. This study has used four different sources: the Bureau of Labor Statistics triennial surveys of hospital workers, 1957-1975; public use samples from the 1960 and 1970 U.S. censuses; annual surveys of hospitals conducted by the American Hospital Association, 1970-1975; and annual surveys of hospital workers' wage scales conducted by the Vanderbilt University Personnel Department, 1970-1977.

Each data base is suited for a particular type of analysis and each provides a unique contribution to understanding hospital wage structures and trends. At the same time, findings of the empirical analyses in chapters 3 through 6 tend to be mutually supportive and produce some consistent themes. The strength of conclusions based on a single parameter estimate is frequently limited by underlying assumptions and potential errors in data or specification. However, when independently performed tests on different data bases arrive at the same general finding, confidence in the results increases enormously. Because each empirical chapter ends with a conclusions and implications section, we do not repeat all of the specifics. Instead, our summary and implications discussions emphasize the common themes from all of the empirical chapters.

Summary of Findings

One of our more important results is largely descriptive, having to do with trends in real wages of hospital workers over the periods studies. The conventional wisdom prior to the mid-1960s was that hospitals employed many low-skilled, low-paid workers and were often "employers of last resort" for those who had difficulty in finding and holding jobs. New revenues generated by the Medicare and Medicaid programs were accompanied by increases in hospital average wages and overall labor expenses during the late 1960s and early 1970s. The upward trend in real hospital wages during this period gave rise to the philanthropic wage hypothesis and theories of hospital inefficiency in response to the infusion of funds from cost-based reimbursement.

It is essential to remember, however, that neither the hospital product nor the composition of the hospital labor force remained constant during this period. Our evidence indicates that, relative to other industry reference groups, worker quality in hospitals increased considerably between 1960 and 1970; there was an upgrading of the hospital work force relative to those in all reference industries evaluated. Quality-adjusted wages of hospital employees, in many instances, remained below comparable wages of reference industry employees. More specifically, relative to male employees in other industries, male hospital employees were still underpaid in 1970. Relative wages of female hospital employees were more favorable although they still earned about 15 percent less than female "manorial" industry workers in 1970.

Further, our evidence indicates that occupation-specific real wages of hospital employees peaked around 1972, and in many cases declined thereafter. Thus while the philanthropic wage hypothesis may have seemed to be a plausible theory to explain trends occurring during a relatively brief span of years following the introduction of Medicare and Medicaid, we reject it as a systematic explanation of hospital wage-setting practices. There is no evidence to suggest that hospital employees are overpaid; indeed, taking increases in worker quality into consideration, hospitals probably should still be regarded as relatively low-paying employers.

These findings might be viewed as justification for a lack of concern about identifying determinants of increases in real hospital wages. However, it is important to identify exogenous influences because of their portent for the future. Our evidence indicates that, historically, both supply- and demand-side factors have had impacts on hospital wage growth. The most important demand-side factors have been the growth of third-party reimbursement and real personal per capita income. But the rapid growth of reimbursement, in terms of persons covered and levels of benefits under private and public health insurance programs, occurred primarily during the 1960s. During the 1970s insurance coverage growth tapered off as almost universal coverage was achieved. Consequently, as is shown rather clearly in analysis of data pertaining to the 1970s (see chapter 5), the influence of third-party reimbursement on hospital wages has diminished in importance. Similarly, compared to the 1960s, increases in real per capita income have been quite modest in the 1970s. It is worth reemphasizing that hospital workers' real wages began to rise rapidly during the prosperous early 1960s before the introduction of Medicare and Medicaid. When (and if) large real income gains are realized in the future, this factor may again become an important hospital wage determinant.

Our findings on the supply-side are more provocative. One unexpected result was the lack of influence of labor market tightness, as indicated by area unemployment rates, on hospital employees' wages. This factor was examined in three separate chapters with mixed results. In a few instances, the expected negative parameter estimate was obtained, but more often it was positive or near zero. This suggests that there are forces at work affecting hospital wage determination that we do not fully understand. As is often the case in empirical research, analyses produce as many questions as answers. Our findings on the effects of unemployment are a good example of this point.

The effects of minimum wage laws on wage rates in hospitals are clearly of policy relevance, especially because hospitals employ a relatively high proportion of low-wage workers, and periodic increases in minimum wages appear to be institutionalized. In chapter 3's empirical analysis we found the expected positive impact of minimum wage laws on hospital workers' wages. The effect is realized not only on low-wage workers but on more highly paid ones as well. Associated elasticities range from 0.03 to 0.15 in chapter 4. Additional empirical work on this topic did not support (nor refute) this finding; but for reasons specified in chapter 4, we believe that the evaluation in chapter 3 merits more confidence. Implications of the impact of minimum wage laws pertain not only to wages but also to hospital production functions. Hospitals are faced with many choices of providing certain nonprofessional services (housekeeping, laundry, and so on) directly or on a contract basis. One expects such choices to be influenced by prevailing wage scales, especially for low-skilled workers.

One of our most consistent and important empirical findings pertains to the effects of unions on hospital employees' wages. These findings are worth reviewing in some detail. Our first indication of union influence came from the analysis in chapter 3 of BLS data on wages in specific occupations. Our estimates indicated substantial union impacts. A change from no hospital union coverage in an SMSA to universal (100 percent) coverage is estimated to boost wages from 4 to 18 percent on average. In terms of the degree of estimated impact, transcribing machine and switchboard operators are at the low end; RNs are midrange (with impacts in the 6 to 7 percent range); and LPNs, medical technologists, and aides-orderlies are at the high end.

The analysis in chapter 4, of state average wages computed from 1970 census data indicated that the proportions of hospitals with collective bargaining agreements and with work stoppages (for example, strikes) have a positive impact on average wage rates in hospitals. Coefficients on the collective bargaining variable imply union impacts on wages in the 13 to 28 percent range, somewhat higher than our estimates in chapter 3. The proportion of hospitals which had received requests from unions for recognition as a collective bargaining agent, however, exhibited no impact on wages. We have interpreted this third variable as a measure of union threat effects and conclude that, at least in the hospital industry, such effects on wages are not consequential.[1]

The findings in chapter 5 on mean hospital employee earnings computed on an individual hospital basis from AHA data are very consistent with the results in chapter 4. Parameter estimates from the regressions in chapter 5 imply that the combined effect on a hospital of both a union and a strike would be to increase average wages 11 to 14 percent. Again, the analysis indicated no effect of requests for collective bargaining recognition.

Chapter 6 added some descriptive evidence on union influence on hospital wages from examination of Vanderbilt University data on wage scales in specific occupations in large hospitals. Among the occupations examined, union growth has not been especially rapid in the mid-1970s. In housekeeping and non-RN nursing occupations, the growth rate was about 1 percent per year. Roughly 24 percent of these employees were unionized in 1977. In RN nursing occupations, the percent unionized was generally less than 10 percent in 1973, but more than doubled over the 1973 to 1977 period. Wage scales of unionized employees were consistently above those of their nonunion counterparts in the same occupations, frequently by as much as 20 percent. We found that unions tend to have a substantial once-and-for-all effect, but that differences in real wage scales between unionized and nonunionized occupations tend to diminish over time.

The rapid increase in hospital costs throughout the 1960s and 1970s has led to the introduction of a number of regulatory programs specifically designed to temper inflation in this sector. Among the most important forms of hospital regulation are capital expenditures-facilities regulation, revenue-cost regulation, and utilization review. Regulatory efforts have largely been at the state level or conducted by Blue Cross plans. An important exception is the Nixon Administration's Economic Stabilization Program (ESP), which was operated nationally during 1971-1974. Clearly such programs may have multifaceted effects, and effects on real hourly wages and annual earnings of hospital workers constitute only a subset at most. For this reason, our empirical analysis of hospital regulation in chapter 5 and, to a limited extent in chapter 6, can only be viewed as a partial assessment of regulatory effects. Yet at the same time estimates of the effect of regulation on real wages and earnings have an important place in any overall evaluation of hospital costs.

In chapter 5, we found no evidence that state prospective reimbursement programs have depressed real annual earnings of hospital employees. Results on ESP and capital-facilities regulation, however, did indicate a restraining influence on hospital wage rates. Evidence on effects of ESP in chapter 5 comes from our descriptive tables rather than from our regression analysis. After rising through 1972, real earnings fell in 1973 and 1974. Although there was some catching up in 1975, hospital workers were still worse off overall in 1975 than in 1972. Descriptive evidence from the Vanderbilt surveys, presented for a variety of occupations, generally show that 1972 was the peak year in terms of real hospital wages. Although there was a substantial rise in money wages after the post-ESP period, workers did not regain their financial positions in real terms. We are reluctant to attribute all post-1971 wage patterns in the Vanderbilt survey data to ESP, but it is reasonable to conclude that ESP played some role. It is worth noting that *Employment and Earnings* (E&E) estimates of mean hourly wages of hospital workers indicate a substantial rise in 1977, not reflected in the Vanderbilt estimates. Yet, with this exception, the series are basically consistent.

Comprehensive certificate-of-need programs that cover bed additions and many other changes in hospital facilities-services were found in chapter 5 to have slightly negative impacts on real earnings, presumably through the effects of such programs on labor mix. Both Section 1122 and Blue Cross Planning Agency

Approval programs were also shown to depress earnings of hospital employees. For Section 1122, the coefficients imply sizable reductions, around 10 to 12 percent.

Implications

Several general policy implications emerge from this study. The following sections describe the most important ones.

Trends in Real Hospital Wages

Hospitals are one of the more labor-intensive industries. While the proportion of total hospital expenditures devoted to labor has decreased in the 1970s, it remains near the 60 percent level on average. In view of the large share of labor costs in total costs, any effective hospital cost containment strategy must monitor labor costs. Yet if one is looking for a culprit as the dominant force underlying hospital cost inflation during the 1970s, it is inappropriate to ascribe a major role to inflation in hospital wage rates. Gauged in terms of wage rates as such, hospital employees have not kept pace with inflation during the 1970s. In fact, as seen in chapter 1, wage patterns in the hospital sector have closely resembled those in other sectors of the U.S. economy. This is in sharp contrast to the 1960s, a decade in which real wages of hospital employees rose both absolutely and relative to employees in other industries. The hospital labor force may be a convenient target for antiinflation policies, but a strict wage control policy, at least in view of data presented in this book, is subject to question on grounds of equity.

The plight of the hospital worker is most evident from the Vanderbilt survey data, which show declines in real minimum and maximum wage rates for specific occupations. It must be emphasized that these rates probably do not reveal the wage progression of the typical hospital employee because there is mobility within and between job classifications. This factor and secular trends in job upgrading are likely reasons for the differences, for example, between the Vanderbilt and the E&E series presented in chapter 1. Yet the Vanderbilt survey evidence does certainly imply that new job entrants into the hospital field do not reap the financial benefits that their counterparts enjoyed half a decade or so ago.

That times change would seem to be so obvious as not to merit mention, but there are numerous statements in the health policy literature to the effect that hospital wages in most job categories have caught up with or surpassed wages of employees in comparable jobs in other industries.[2] Such statements tend to be accompanied by data series describing the growth in hospital wages that end in 1972. Our work suggests that it is wise to extend the series further before making policy inferences about hospital wage inflation.

An important element of any form of revenue-cost regulation, both at the state as well as programs currently being contemplated at the federal level, involves the treatment of wages. Should there be wage pass throughs, and if so, for which types of workers? It has sometimes been argued (see Feldstein 1979) that failure to include wage restraints in a rate regulation program leaves the door open for substantial hospital wage increases. Throughout most of the 1970s, hospital wages have been uncontrolled in the vast majority of states; and real wages have not risen to any meaningful extent, and we have documented some real wage decreases. Whether hospital regulatory arrangements should be implemented involves a number of considerations beyond the scope of this study. But judging from the wage trends documented in our study, the rationale for general wage controls over hospital employees at the present time is weak at best. There is greater justification for selective government intervention, such as over wage settlements established via collective bargaining. We consider this issue further in subsequent sections.

Hospital Wage-Scale Compression

Some evidence is presented in this book suggesting a compression in wage scales—low-skilled hospital employees have made some gains relative to their high-skilled counterparts. Compression could reflect a number of developments: tightening labor markets for low-skilled workers; increased numbers of graduates from the specialized training programs (such as professional nursing and medical technology); greater extent of collective bargaining activity in low-skilled categories; increases in the real minimum wage; and low-wage exceptions under various revenue—cost regulation programs. Unfortunately, our empirical studies do not allow one to choose among these potential reasons. But at the same time, the compression has not been very large.

To sort out the reasons for wage compression seems deceptively simple at first glance, but spillovers make this task difficult. For example, we have found that minimum-wage legislation affects wages in a great number of skill classes, not just those around the minimum. This widespread effect is predicted by the neoclassical model or by a model which assumes that hospitals seek to maintain a reasonably fixed occupational wage structure. Second, in several cases, our estimates are too imprecise to permit inferences about determinants of relative hospital wages. The unexpectedly positive unemployment rate parameters in our wage regressions force us to be cautious about making definitive statements about the role of tightening labor markets for the economy as a whole. The unexplained positive parameters on measures of output of state training programs in certain skilled hospital occupations preclude our making statements about the effect of expanded training programs on hospital wages. Although some hospital rate regulatory programs exempt low-wage employees, the dependent variable in our chapter on regulation is insufficiently refined to ever pick up any exemption effects on hospital wage structure.

To the extent that policymakers are concerned about the effects of antiinflation strategies on low-wage workers, wage compression in the hospital industry might be viewed as desirable, especially in light of the recent real wage declines in this industry. Our inability to isolate specific causes for this compression should mitigate any optimism, however, because we cannot with any degree of confidence predict how specific hospital cost containment strategies would affect low-wage workers relative to higher paid hospital employees.

Worker Quality

We have documented a definite upgrading in the labor force during the decade of the 1960s, both in absolute terms and relative to other industries. As *quality* is defined, not all of the upgrading is necessarily reflected in higher productivity. Our index of labor quality reflects employer willingness to pay for specific employee attributes. In some instances, willingness to pay unquestionably reflects tastes shared in common by a large group of employers, both in and outside the hospital sector, and may well be unrelated to labor productivity, turnover, or any other dimension of efficiency.

Unfortunately, it is not now possible to precisely gauge changes in hospital work-force composition, given the paucity of data on the quantities of various types of labor employed. The Current Population Surveys, conducted on a regular basis by the U.S. Census Bureau, are one source of such data; but, given the relatively small sample size of this source, analysis of these data would necessarily be much more limited than in chapter 4. The 1980 census of population will provide another opportunity to examine changes in work-force composition and its determinants. Lacking evidence from this source at the present time but armed with evidence from sources presented in this book, one is reasonably safe in concluding that comparatively little upgrading has occurred in the hospital sector during the 1970s, both in absolute terms and relative to other industries.

Why did the upgrading observed during the 1960s occur? And can we expect it to have continued? First, it should be emphasized that this trend reflects much more than qualitative changes in the U.S. work force as a whole, since the hospital work force changed relative to those in other industries. In effect, the reference groups serve as controls for examining this type of phenomenon. One is tempted to conclude on the basis of the descriptive analysis that the growth in both third-party coverage and real personal per capita income is responsible, at least in large part. Although this explanation should not be rejected, the single-year regressions in chapter 4 do not show consistently positive effects of reimbursement and per capita income on hospital work-force quality. Perhaps introduction of Medicare and Medicaid, coupled with rising per capita income, produced a shock effect that cannot be captured by regression analysis of single cross sections.[3]

While there is still some uncertainty as to the causes of variations in hospital work-force composition, the notion that hospitals used their newly found third-party revenue to upgrade their work forces seems to us a great deal more plausible than the view that hospitals used such funds to pay their employees economic rents. To some extent, a "better" work force benefits hospital employers in terms of reduced costs of on-the-job training and turnover. In any case, our analysis clearly indicates that the philanthropic wage hypothesis has little or no validity as an explanation for recent hospital wage trends. Moreover, to the extent that the composition is changing, hospitals will become less dependable employers of last resort. Thus manpower policies aimed at reducing unemployment rates among the disadvantaged will increasingly have to rely on other industries.

Some changes in work-force composition are attributable to technological change, which in turn is a response to many of the exogenous factors included in our regressions. Technological change in most industries is likely to bring about some substitution of nonlabor for labor inputs. This is seldom true for hospitals, where technological change typically creates demands for skilled labor to operate and maintain newly developed equipment.

Although it seems natural that hospital worker "quality" should increase with technological advances, one ought to examine this tendency more closely. Many, if not most, of the services performed in hospitals are not technologically intensive but involve relatively simple acts of caring for the ill and disabled. Several experts have expressed the view that a technological orientation may benefit some patients but tends to dehumanize hospital care to the detriment of the majority of patients. Lengthy discussion of this issue would take us far afield of our topic. It may be useful in the present context, however, to emphasize that hospital technological advances create not only capital expenditures but also added labor expenses as well. Our evidence on recent regulatory program impacts on hospital wage rates supports this view. Programs designed to control hospital capital expenditures, particularly those that pay close attention to equipment purchases and expansion of services, tend to have a negative effect on average wages.[4] Thus the debate over costs and benefits of alternative styles of hospital care ought to include the effect of technological intensity on employee mix and average wages.

Not all work-force upgrading in hospitals is attributable to changing employee mix in response to technological change. Within the nursing profession, for example, there has been a movement for several years promoting greater educational attainments for RNs, primarily in terms of substituting baccalaureate degrees for nursing diplomas. Whether this kind of upgrading is necessary to keep up with technological advances is uncertain and subject to some controversy. However, to the extent that increased educational attainments affect average nursing wages without offsetting effects on productivity, this trend is an identifiable source of increase in hospital costs.

Worker Protectionism

Developments on the supply side, especially increased minimum wages and unionization, have unquestionably boosted hospital employees' wages. Although such policies as raising the minimum wage and extending protection to employee groups who wish to organize collectively *may* benefit some hospital employees, these policies are inflationary.[5] Therefore in evaluating the distributional impacts of minimum wages and other legislation designed to assist the poor or near-poor worker, policymakers ought to consider the additional effects of hospital cost and price increases generated by such policies.

Occupations often seek legislation granting them exclusive "franchises" over specific spheres of activity, arguing that licenses will protect the consumer from unscrupulous and inadequately trained suppliers. Whether licensure results in improved quality on the average, or at least quality above some acceptable minimum, is subject to considerable debate. Recently, licensure has been questioned increasingly on antitrust grounds.

This study provides no estimates of the impact of various types of health occupation licensure on the quality of services rendered. However, estimates reported in chapter 3 clearly indicate that licensure (mandatory licensure in the case of nursing) has raised real wages of personnel in the licensed occupations, and the estimated effects are by no means trivial, especially in the case of medical technologists. Although it is unlikely that states will return to permissive licensure of nursing personnel, many states have not yet enacted licensure laws for such health occupations as medical technologists. In listening to testimony by various professions concerning the public benefits to be derived from licensure, legislators should also keep in mind that there are definite private financial benefits to persons in licensed professions as well.

In considering the future of the hospital labor force, it is clear that unionization is likely to be of major importance. While this study provides evidence from a variety of sources to support this conclusion, there are a number of questions that remain unanswered. Although unions gained entry into some hospitals decades ago, it is appropriate to view 1974, the year in which the Taft-Hartley Act was extended to include hospitals within the jurisdiction of collective bargaining legislation, as the year in which the concept of hospital unions gains full legitimacy. As of this writing, there are insufficient data available to fully describe the growth of unions in hospitals or, indeed, whether it is legitimate to call hospital union growth a movement. Our most recent evidence, obtained from the American Hospital Association surveys, indicates that the growth rate since 1974 has not been especially rapid; as of 1977, the vast majority of hospitals had no union representation. Yet we anticipate that this growth will continue in the foreseeable future. Although we cannot predict how far unionization will penetrate into the hospital labor force, there can be no doubt that this is a trend that bears close attention by policymakers. Given its implications for hospital cost inflation, intervention by government to control the rate or nature of union growth may be warranted.

All of our evidence indicates that unions exert a positive and important impact on hospital wage rates and service costs. Beyond this general conclusion, we are uncertain of the specific nature of union impact. One important issue is the relative magnitude of the once-and-for-all effect versus the long-term effect. Our evidence indicates primarily that the once-and-for-all effect dominates, and that union/nonunion real wage differences tend to diminish over time. Our data to support this conclusion are scanty, however, and ought to be replicated with more complete evidence covering longer time periods and more hospitals, occupations, and employees.

One important factor omitted from our analysis is the amount, growth, and union influence on fringe benefits. For several reasons, including demographic composition of employees and industry structure, we might expect the growth and development of fringes in the hospital industry to follow a different course from other industries. In any case, we have no evidence of union effects on fringe benefits; if such effects are positive, our estimates of union impact on hospital employee wages may understate the effect on total employee compensation to an unknown degree.

Another more subtle but equally as important potential effect of unions is on hospital production functions and styles of care. In most industries, where outputs are less heterogeneous, one can reasonably well predict the consequences of increasing labor costs due to union influence on wages, fringe benefits, and working conditions. But in the case of the hospital industry, one cannot make such predictions with confidence. Many of the employees in hospital bargaining units are professionals, including nurses, who bring at least some issues to the bargaining table that have ramifications for service delivery. In addition, collective bargaining may influence decisions on what nonprofessional services are offered and whether to provide them directly or on a contract basis. As an example, potential or actual union coverage may convince a hospital to obtain laundry services on a contract basis. At present, these are pure speculations; in future research they may be formalized into hypotheses for empirical analysis.[6] We are convinced, however, that the influence of unions on hospital performance may extend far beyond an upward impact on wage rates.

Monopsony

At the other extreme from the notion that hospitals are philanthropic wage setters is the monopsony hypothesis. Typically, monopsonies arise when a factor (1) is specialized, with few potential substitutes, and (2) is immobile. Although the issue has interested researchers, there are also policy implications in that minimum wage legislation and legislation favorable to collective bargaining are often rationalized on grounds that employers exploit (that is, exercise monopsony power over) employees and government must provide the offsetting influence.

Although tests of monopsony power in the hospital field have been applied to hospital workers as a whole (see Davis 1973), on conceptual grounds, it makes considerably more sense to focus on the more specialized hospital occupations, such as professional nursing. It is generally argued that monopsony power is more likely to occur in communities in which hospital output (and hence input employment) is highly concentrated, and we agree. Concentration lowers the costs of collusion among hospital employers. As an empirical matter, however, various concentration measures are closely related to city size (see appendix D). Hence, that lower RN wages are observed in relatively small cities with a highly concentrated hospital sector may only mean that prices of goods and services are lower there; and the relationship between concentration and wages may well be a spurious one. In our view, progress will not be made by researchers on the monopsony issue until more direct measures of employer collusion are obtained. In the meantime, we believe that any conclusions about hospitals' use of monopsony power are conjectures at best.

Regulation

This study represents an initial attempt to focus on hospital regulation as it applies to labor markets. Some impacts have been detected, but there is much more to be learned. For example, what impact is revenue-cost regulation likely to have on the growth of hospital unions; and once hospital employees are organized, does this type of regulation affect the bargaining process and/or outcomes? A more formative question is should hospitals be placed at risk for increased wages under revenue-cost regulation? And if so, under which circumstances? Should wages for certain types of hospital employees be exempt from regulation?

If wages are exogenous to the individual hospital, one might be tempted to say wages should be exempt. Yet matters are not nearly so simple, since wage rates may be exogenous to the hospital but endogenous to a larger market area under the purview of the regulatory authority. Certainly our empirical evidence indicates that wages paid hospital employees have been different from those paid comparable employees in other industries. Most wages are not fixed to the local hospital industry in the sense that if hospitals do not pay the going (nonhospital) rate they will lose their workers. Hence, although regulation of hospital wages may place hospitals at some competitive disadvantage if other industries remain unregulated, there is sufficient play in the system to allow hospitals to conduct their daily activities. On the other hand, because hospital workers' real wages have not increased in recent years, regulatory emphasis on controlling wages may be misplaced from the vantage point of equity.

Changes in employee mix may be constrained indirectly by limiting the types of hospital services which third parties are allowed to finance. For example, the trend toward worker upgrading may be slowed by effective regulation of hospital equipment purchases and implementation of sophisticated new medical procedures. It is important to recognize that such regulations have the potential of affecting demands for different types of labor, particularly for workers with hospital-specific skills. Yet, as we have said, hospital work-force upgrading seems to be slowing, and the case for restraints on employee mix changes is weaker than it might have been a decade ago.

There has been a considerable amount of regulatory activity in the hospital sector in the 1970s, relatively little of which has been directed specifically at the hospital work force. Yet it is likely that hospital labor will have felt some of the consequences, and only a fraction of potential effects have been considered in this study. Because labor commands such a high proportion of hospital expenditures, it would be foolish not to include labor impacts in planning regulatory strategies, regardless of whether such strategies are intended to influence labor mix or costs. Similarly, researchers concerned with measuring regulatory effects on hospitals would be remiss to ignore indirect effects on the hospital work force. As advances on the regulatory front continue into the 1980s, and such advances seem unstoppable at this writing, we hope that those responsible for implementation will be astute enough to realize that literally millions of hospital workers are likely to be affected.

Notes

1. Our findings on the collective bargaining recognition variable should be contrasted with those in our companion study, Sloan and Steinwald (forthcoming, 1980). Using AHA data on individual hospitals over 1970 to 1975, we obtained positive and significant parameter estimates on a collective bargaining recognition variable in total hospital cost and labor cost regressions. The most likely source of the discrepancy is that labor costs in the companion study included the monetary value of fringe benefits. Fringe benefit costs have, in fact, been increasing at a more rapid pace during the 1970s than other labor and nonlabor hospital costs (American Hospital Association 1978). Thus if there is a

threat effect of unionization, it may be realized in nonwage expenditures designed to forestall union entry into hospitals.

2. Three recent works are Hughes et al. (1978), Feldstein and Taylor (1977), and Fuchs (1976). Feldstein and Taylor's wage series ends with 1972. Fuchs' analysis, based on U.S. census data, is for 1960 and 1970. In most research one can legitimately be unconcerned about a gap of a few years between the end point of the data series and the publication date. However, the issue of hospital wage trends in the 1970s appears to be one case where the gap can contribute to misleading results.

3. A similar pattern emerges from empirical analysis by Davis (forthcoming, 1973).

4. However, in our companion study (Sloan and Steinwald, forthcoming, 1980) we found no effect of such programs on total and labor costs per admission or adjusted patient day. The discrepancy may be due to different specifications or, in the companion study, a negative influence on average wages may be offset by added costs elsewhere not captured in the present analysis. In any case, given the discrepancy, we are unwilling to emphasize chapter 5's results pertaining to regulation.

5. The inflationary effect of collective bargaining efforts is more evident when hospital costs are the dependent variables. See Sloan and Steinwald (forthcoming, 1980).

6. The authors are currently engaged in further research on union influence on hospital behavior under Grant No. 18-P-97090/4-01 from the Health Care Financing Administration to Vanderbilt University.

Appendixes

Appendix A
Area Price Indexes

Introduction

All monetarily expressed variables have been deflated by an area price index. Since no official area index exists, it has been necessary to construct indexes for each of our empirical chapters (chapters 3 through 6). The precise needs of each chapter differ; so it has been necessary to construct a separate index for each. Chapter 3 requires an area price index for large cities, 1960-1975. In chapter 4, we had to work with the constraint that the smallest geographical unit identified on our U.S. Census Public Use tapes is the state, and, therefore, a state price index has been used. In chapters 5 and 6, area price information was needed for specific locations for the 1970s.

To describe all indexes in detail would take us far afield. It is possible for readers to gain the "flavor" by describing the construction of one index in detail; the remainder of this appendix discusses the one in chapter 5. It is worth emphasizing that the indexes used in chapters 3, 5, and 6 are expressed in 1972 dollars. For the state price index, in chapter 4, it was necessary to select a representative SMSA for all SMSAs in the state; and the nonmetropolitan index for the census area (Northeast, North Central, South, or West) stands for all nonmetropolitan areas in a given state. The chapter 4 price index is in 1960 dollars. Finally, some of the assignments of index values to areas with missing data are admittedly arbitrary.

Methodology for the Area Price
Index in Chapter 5

Step 1: Record cost of living (COL) index data for available metropolitan areas for 1972, using U.S. Bureau of Labor Statistics (BLS) data for each area.[1] Cost of living is taken for an intermediate budget family of four (1972 metropolitan average = 1.00).

Step 2: For areas without corresponding BLS metropolitan area COL data, the following assignment procedure was used (see table A-1);

    1. For metropolitan areas, data pertaining to nearby metropolitan areas of similar size, for which BLS COL data were available, were assigned.

    2. For nonmetropolitan areas, BLS data pertaining to nonmetropolitan areas by census region (Northeast, South, Midwest, West) were assigned.

Step 3: COL index values for years other than 1972 were adjusted according to

Table A-1

Cost of Living Data Assignments for Nonmetropolitan Areas and for Metropolitan Areas without Bureau of Labor Statistics Data Available, by State

State	Nonmetropolitan[a]	Metropolitan[b]
Alabama	South	Atlanta, Ga.
Alaska	Anchorage[c]	Anchorage, Alas.
Arizona	West	Bakersfield, Calif.
Arkansas	South	Baton Rouge, La.
California	West	Bakersfield, Calif.
Colorado	West	Denver, Colo.
Connecticut	Northeast	Hartford, Conn.
Delaware	South	Philadelphia, Pa.
Florida	South	Orlando, Fla.
Georgia	South	Atlanta, Ga.
Hawaii	Honolulu[e]	Honolulu, Haw.
Idaho	West	Denver, Colo.
Illinois	Midwest	Champaign-Urbana, Ill.
Indiana	Midwest	Indianapolis, Ind.
Iowa	Midwest	Cedar Rapids, Iowa
Kansas	Midwest	Wichita, Kans.
Kentucky	South	Nashville, Tenn.
Louisiana	South	Baton Rouge, La.
Maine	Northeast	Portland, Me.
Maryland	South	Baltimore, Md.
Massachusetts	Northeast	Boston, Mass.
Michigan	Midwest	Detroit, Mich.
Minnesota	Midwest	Minneapolis-St. Paul, Minn.
Mississippi	South	Baton Rouge, La.
Missouri	South	Kansas City, Mo.
Montana	West	Seattle-Everett, Wash.
Nebraska	West	Cedar Rapids, Iowa
Nevada	West	Bakersfield, Calif.
New Hampshire	Northeast	Portland, Me.
New Jersey	Northeast	Philadelphia, Pa.
New Mexico	West	Denver, Colo.
New York	Northeast	Buffalo, N.Y.
North Carolina	South	Durham, N.C.
North Dakota	Midwest	Minneapolis-St. Paul, Minn.
Ohio	Midwest	Dayton, Ohio
Oklahoma	South	Dallas, Tex.
Oregon	West	Seattle-Everett, Wash.
Pennsylvania	Northeast	Lancaster, Pa.
Rhode Island	Northeast	Boston, Mass.
South Carolina	South	Atlanta, Ga.
South Dakota	Midwest	Minneapolis-St. Paul, Minn.
Tennessee	South	Nashville, Tenn.
Texas	South	Austin, Tex.
Utah	West	Denver, Colo.
Vermont	Northeast	Portland, Me.
Virginia	South	Durham, N.C.
Washington	West	Seattle-Everett, Wash.
Washington, D.C.	—	d

Table A-1 *(continued)*

State	Nonmetropolitan[a]	Metropolitan[b]
West Virginia	South	Durham, N.C.
Wisconsin	Midwest	Green Bay, Wisc.
Wyoming	West	Bakersfield, Cal.

[a]Nonmetropolitan cost of living index values were assigned by census area (Northeast, South, North Central, or West).

[b]Metropolitan cost of living index values were assigned as shown for all metropolitan areas in the state for which BLS data were unavailable.

[c]Anchorage SMSA data assigned to all of Alaska.

[d]District of Columbia metropolitan area data available.

[e]Honolulu SMSA data assigned to all of Hawaii.

changes in SMSA-specific Consumer Price Index values. Years prior to 1972 were adjusted downward and years after 1972 were adjusted upward. The result is an index for use in converting variables measured in nominal dollars to real terms, correcting for interarea variations in price levels. National means of the price index series used to express the index in 1972 dollars are as follows:

1969:	0.0876
1970:	0.928
1971:	0.968
1972:	1.000
1973:	1.062
1974:	1.179
1975:	1.287

Note

1. Direct data are available for the following SMSAs: Boston, Mass.; Buffalo, N.Y.; Hartford, Conn.; Lancaster, Pa.; New York-Northeastern N.J.; Philadelphia, Pa.-N.J.; Pittsburgh, Pa.; Portland, Me.; Cedar Rapids, Iowa; Champaign-Urbana, Ill.; Chicago, Ill.-Northwestern Ind.; Cincinnati, Ohio-Ky.-Ind.; Cleveland, Ohio; Dayton, Ohio; Detroit, Mich.; Green Bay, Wisc.; Indianapolis, Ind.; Kansas City, Mo.-Kans.; Milwaukee, Wisc.; Minneapolis-St. Paul, Minn.; St. Louis, Mo.-Ill.; Wichita, Kans.; Atlanta, Ga.; Austin, Tex.; Baltimore, Md.; Baton Rouge, La.; Dallas, Tex.; Durham, N.C.; Houston, Tex.; Nashville, Tenn.; Orlando, Fla.; Washington, D.C.-Md.-Va.; Bakersfield, Cal.; Denver, Colo.; Los Angeles-Long Beach, Cal.; San Diego, Cal.; San Francisco-Oakland, Cal.; Seattle-Everett, Wash.; Honolulu, Haw.; and Anchorage, Alaska. See Sloan and Steinwald (forthcoming, 1980) for area definitions and list.

Appendix B
Data Sources for
Chapter 3

Dependent Variables

Wage data have been obtained from *Industry Wage Surveys: Hospitals*, published every three years by the U.S. Bureau of Labor Statistics (BLS Bulletin no. 1294, 1409, 1553, 1688, 1829, and 1949). Wage data for 1957, coded but not used, are available from Bulletin no. 1210.

Explanatory Variables

1. *Occupation-specific wages for the SMSA as a whole (AWAGE).* Wage data for SMSAs included in BLS hospital surveys have been coded for transcribing machine operators, switchboard operators, and porters-maids. When wage data on class A and B switchboard operators were provided, we took class B. Wages for transcribing machine and switchboard operators are for female employees. Those for porters-maids are for men and women. When male and female wages are listed separately, we have used the male-female proportions for porters and maids in hospitals in the SMSA and year as weights. Wage data are published by the BLS as *Industry Wage Surveys* (BLS Bulletin no. 1285-83, 1385-82, 1530-87, 1660-91, and individual numbers in the 1850 series for 1975).

2. *Unemployment rates by "labor area" (UN).* The Bureau of Labor Statistics publishes annual data on unemployment rates in 150 major labor areas (cities) in the *Employment and Training Report of the President* (formerly *Manpower Report of the President*). Pre- and post-1970 unemployment data are not completely comparable. Fortunately, there is some overlap in the unemployment series to permit us to compute city-specific adjustment factors. The conversion process puts pre-1970 unemployment rates in post-1970 terms.

3. *State and federal minimum wages (MWAGE).* A minimum wage series by state has been constructed from the following sources: U.S. Department of Labor, Wage Standards Administration, *Annual Digests of State and Federal Labor Legislation*; U.S. Department of Labor, Women's Bureau, *State Minimum Wage Laws* (7/1/55, 7/1/58, 1/1/60, 6/1/62, 7/1/63, 1/1/65, 4/66); U.S. Department of Labor, Bureau of Labor Standards, *Brief Summary of State Minimum Wage Laws* (8/64 and 1/65); U.S. Department of Labor, Wage Standards Administration, *Minimum Wage Legislation,* 1967 (no. 313); U.S. Department of Labor, Report to Congress, *A Study to Measure the Effects of*

*the Minimum Wage and Maximum Hours Standards of the Fair Labor Standards
Act,* January 1967, processed. In cases when both federal and state laws apply,
we have taken the higher of the two. Construction of MWAGE has involved a
number of sources, and to describe all necessary assumptions would take a
number of pages; we have assembled minimum wage source material in a
notebook, which interested researchers in this area may wish to consult.

4. *Extent of unionization in hospitals by SMSA (UNION).* This variable and
the method of construction are described in chapter 3 and appendix C. Data
come from BLS Bulletin no. 1409, 1553, 1668, and 1949.

5. *State licensure of RNs, LPNs, and medical technologists (MLC).* Licensure applies only to three occupations in chapter 3. Since RNs and LPNs
were licensed in all states throughout the observational period, the licensure
variable for these two groups is based on the mandatory versus permissive
distinction. For medical technologists, MLC simply distinguishes between states
with and without licensure. Our licensure variables are based on these sources:
U.S. Health Manpower Commission (1967); U.S. Bureau of Labor Statistics and
U.S. Department of Health, Education, and Welfare, *State Licensing of Health
Occupations,* 1968 (PHS Publication no. 1758); and annual issues of the
American Nurses Association, *Facts About Nursing.*

6. *Number of graduates in professional and practical nursing by state per
1,000 state population (RNGRAD, LPNGRAD, and TCGRAD).* Unfortunately,
data on the number of graduates for these three occupations are only available at
the state level. Data on nursing graduates, both RN and LPN, come from *Facts
About Nursing,* a publication of the American Nurses Association. The number
of graduates of medical technology programs comes from two sources. For 1966
and before, state estimates have been constructed from data on individual
programs provided in education number(s) of the *Journal of the American
Medical Association.* Since 1966, data come from various editions of *Health
Resources Statistics,* National Center for Health Statistics, U.S. Public Health
Service.

7. *Locational amenities by state (MUR and AUTO).* Homicide and auto
theft data come from U.S. Department of Justice, *Uniform Crime Reports,*
published annually.

8. *Per capita income in the SMSA (INC).* 1975 definitions of SMSAs have
been used (with population weights) to construct SMSA estimates from county
data. Source: Volumes of the American Medical Association's *Distribution of
Physicians* series.

9. *Proportion of hospital expenses covered by private and public third
parties by state (REIM).* The denominator of REIM is total expenditures on
services in nonfederal, short-term general and other special hospitals, available
annually from American Hospital Association and published since 1972 in
Hospital Statistics (earlier data in *Guide Issues,* which appeared as part II of the
August 1 issue of *Hospitals*). For the numerator, we have derived an estimate of

third-party payor expenditures on hospital services; the numerator consists of expenditures by Blue Cross and commercial insurers and Medicare and Medicaid. Separate estimates of Blue Cross and commercial insurance benefit payments to hospitals are unavailable by state. Benefit payments on all types of health services are available from annual issues of the Health Insurance Institute's *Source Books of Health Insurance Data.* National estimates of the proportions of Blue Cross-Blue Shield payments going to hospitals are published annually in the *Social Security Bulletin.* We have applied the national proportion of hospital benefits to total benefits for the year to separate private insurer payments for hospital services from payments for other health services. The Medicare expenditure component represents payments on Medicare Part A, available annually by state (since July 1966). Medicaid payments are state vendor payments for hospital services, published in annual *Statistical Supplements, Social Security Bulletin.* In more recent years, these data are available from publications of the National Center for Social Statistics (for example, *Medicaid Statistics, Public Assistance Statistics*).

10. *Physician and bed availability by SMSA (MD and BEDS).* Nonfederal, office-based physicians per 1,000 population and nonfederal short-term general hospital beds per 1,000 population have been calculated in the same manner as per capita income (aggregated to the SMSA from the county level) and from the same source, the American Medical Association's *Distribution of Physicians* series. See no. 8 in this appendix.

Appendix C
Collective Bargaining
in Hospitals

Since 1966, the Bureau of Labor Statistics has published estimates of the percentage of hospitals in selected SMSAs having collective bargaining agreements covering a majority of their employees. These data are available for the SMSAs listed in the tables in appendix D. Unionization data are given for four broad occupational categories: RNs, other professional and technical, office clerical, and nonprofessional employees. An exception is 1975, as described in chapter 3. We have made adjustments to make the 1975 data as comparable to the earlier years as possible.

All data sources employed in various chapters of this study show that collective bargaining has a significantly positive and meaningful (in terms of estimated elasticities) effect on wages. Thus it is of some interest to know why unionization rates vary among SMSAs and over time.

Table C-1 contains union coverage regressions for each of the four occupational groups. The dependent variable for each group is UNION, which was used as an explanatory variable in the empirical analysis in chapter 3. Separate dependent variables are defined for each of the four broad occupational categories listed here. It is worth emphasizing that the dependent variable refers to the percentage of hospitals having agreements covering the *majority* of employees in a given occupational category.

The first explanatory variable in table C-1 is NAGU, the fraction of nonagricultural employees who are unionized, defined for the state in which the SMSA is located. These data come from *Statistical Abstracts of the United States.* Variables T66, T69, and T72 are dummy variables for the years 1966, 1969, and 1972, respectively, the omitted category being 1975.

Variables STRONGS, STRONGL, and STRONGP identify SMSAs with strong laws supportive of collective bargaining activity. The first two refer to state laws governing collective bargaining in state and local government agencies, respectively. The variables are one if the state has a law requiring state (STRONGS) or local (STRONGL) employers to bargain colectively when employees so request, and the observation refers to government hospitals. The idea for constructing this measure comes from Kochan (1973). Sourcebooks on public sector bargaining laws also used for our analysis are listed in Kochan. The variable STRONGP, which measures the same type of legislation affecting private hospitals, is based on *Iowa Law Review* (1971-1972), updated with Commerce Clearing House citations on collective bargaining legislation. It is one when there is a statute strongly supportive of collective bargaining in private hospitals and the observation refers to private hospitals.

Table C-1
Determinants of Collective Bargaining Activity in Hospitals

Explanatory Variable	Professional Nurses	Other Professional and Technical	Office Clerical	Nonprofessional
NAGU	0.90* (0.26)	0.69* (0.21)	0.58** (0.23)	1.26* (0.27)
STRONGS	0.35* (0.12)	0.16 (0.10)	0.27** (0.11)	0.19 (0.13)
STRONGL	0.075 (0.12)	0.096 (0.096)	0.022 (0.11)	0.049 (0.13)
STRONGP	0.0005 (0.079)	−0.023 (0.060)	−0.13 (0.066)	−0.064 (0.076)
T66	−0.17** (0.08)	−0.18* (0.063)	−0.29* (0.072)	−0.26* (0.082)
T69	−0.088 (0.075)	−0.16* (0.061)	−0.24* (0.069)	−0.26* (0.078)
T72	0.021 (0.069)	−0.13** (0.058)	−0.15** (0.066)	−0.086 (0.075)
CONSTANT	−0.058	0.028	0.17	0.082
	$R^2 = 0.41$ $R^2(C) = 0.38$ $F(7,138) = 13.6*$	$R^2 = 0.29$ $R^2(C) = 0.26$ $F(7,152) = 9.0*$	$R^2 = 0.29$ $R^2(C) = 0.25$ $F(7,154) = 8.9*$	$R^2 = 0.31$ $R^2(C) = 0.28$ $F(7,149) = 9.5*$

Note: Figures in parentheses are standard errors.
*Significant at the 1 percent level (two-tail test); **Significant at the 5 percent level (two-tail test).

The most consistently significant coefficients in table C-1 relate to NAGU and the year dummies. Not surprisingly, when a high proportion of the nonagricultural work force is organized, hospital employees tend to be organized as well. Probably the major reasons for this association are (1) that the necessary expertise for organizing hospital workers is more readily available in highly unionized states, and (2) worker acceptance of the notion of unionization is higher. The year dummies show, not surprisingly, that holding other factors constant, collective bargaining activity has been increasing over time. Judging from the coefficients, increases since 1966 have been most pronounced in the office-clerical and nonprofessional occupational groups. The growth of collective bargaining in professional nursing, according to the table C-1 estimates, was quite slow during the first half of the 1970s. The year dummies account for time-related increases in collective bargaining not explained by NAGU and the STRONG variables.

Variables STRONGS and STRONGL are highly collinear (with simple correlations in excess of 0.8). Thus although the standard errors on STRONGL are large relative to their associated parameter estimates, one should not conclude that laws strongly supportive of collective bargaining in local government agencies have no effect. Rather, in view of the positive and reasonably precise coefficients on STRONGS, it is appropriate to conclude (tentatively) that such laws have an effect on public sector hospitals. On the other hand, the coefficients and associated standard errors on STRONGP suggest no effect.

Appendix D
Measures of Hospital
Concentration

This appendix serves two functions. First, it provides a list of the Standard Metropolitan Statistical Areas (SMSAs) used in the empirical analysis in chapter 3. Tables D-1 and D-2 list the SMSAs for which BLS data are available for at least one of the six years (1960, 1963, 1966, 1969, 1972, and 1975) included in the regressions in chapter 3. Most of these SMSAs were included in the majority of years. Just because an observation on an SMSA was not available for a given year, we did not throw out the SMSA for years for which wage data are available from the BLS.

Second, and more important, tables D-1 and D-2 each give four measures of concentration for 1969, 1972, and 1975. Table D-1 expresses concentration in terms of hospital beds; table D-2 is based on full-time equivalent hospital personnel (FTE) rather than beds. Calculations are based on *Annual Survey of Hospitals* tapes, provided by the American Hospital Association. The four measures in both tables are four-hospital concentration ratio, eight-hospital concentration ratio, Herfindahl index, and entropy index. The four- and eight-hospital measures gauge the percentage of beds of FTEs accounted for, respectively, by the four or eight largest hospitals in the SMSA. These are very standard measures from the industrial organization literature (a specialty within economics). The Herfindahl and entropy indexes are more comprehensive in that the relative size of all hospitals in the community are taken into account. Higher values on the Herfindahl index indicate higher concentration; less negative values on the entropy index indicate the same. The formula for the entropy index is shown in chapter 3.

Several features are notable about the tables. First, all four measures show essentially the same pattern. As a rule, it is probably not worth calculating all four. Second, concentration is inversely related to SMSA size. For example, beds and FTEs are much more concentrated in Chattanooga than in New York City. Third, tables D-1 and D-2 reveal somewhat different trends over 1969-1975. On the whole, using the beds measures, concentration seems to be falling over time. Using FTEs, the patterns are far more irregular. While these differentials imply that one should be concerned about the type of variable used to gauge concentration, we do not know a sufficient amount about concentration determinants to suggest reasons for the differences between the two tables.

Table D-1
Concentration Measures: Beds

SMSA	Four-Hospital Concentration Ratio (%)			Eight-Hospital Concentration Ratio (%)			Herfindahl Index			Entropy Index		
	1969	1972	1975	1969	1972	1975	1969	1972	1975	1969	1972	1975
Atlanta	45.0	35.3	29.9	68.4	56.7	49.0	0.08	0.06	0.05	-2.9	-3.1	-3.4
Baltimore	47.5	43.9	36.9	62.9	58.2	52.7	0.07	0.06	0.05	-3.1	-3.2	-3.3
Boston	23.0	20.2	17.9	37.6	31.8	27.8	0.02	0.02	0.02	-4.2	-4.3	-4.4
Buffalo	55.5	47.4	35.3	70.6	66.0	58.2	0.11	0.08	0.06	-2.7	-2.8	-3.1
Chattanooga	67.5	68.9	62.4	85.8	86.8	81.9	0.18	0.16	0.13	-2.2	-2.2	-2.4
Chicago	24.8	17.7	13.3	59.6	26.2	21.6	0.23	0.02	0.01	-4.4	-4.5	-4.6
Cincinnati	55.7	49.6	43.9	75.7	71.5	68.8	0.14	0.11	0.08	-2.6	-2.7	-2.8
Cleveland	31.6	26.6	27.0	47.9	43.2	42.5	0.05	0.04	0.04	-3.3	-3.5	-3.5
Dallas	43.6	42.1	33.3	59.6	57.7	48.3	0.08	0.07	0.05	-3.3	-3.4	-3.7
Denver	30.3	30.6	31.0	53.1	52.6	52.1	0.05	0.05	0.05	-3.1	-3.1	-3.2
Detroit	33.1	24.5	19.1	45.8	36.6	31.2	0.04	0.03	0.02	-3.8	-4.0	-4.1
Houston	38.7	34.3	29.2	55.7	51.8	45.0	0.05	0.04	0.04	-3.4	-3.6	-3.7
Los Angeles-Long Beach	24.4	18.9	17.4	31.4	31.7	25.3	0.02	0.02	0.01	-4.6	-4.8	-4.8
Memphis	74.3	78.9	72.5	93.5	92.9	86.3	0.18	0.20	0.19	-2.0	-2.0	-2.1
Miami	46.5	39.1	32.0	66.4	57.6	49.3	0.09	0.07	0.05	-2.8	-3.0	-3.3
Milwaukee	39.4	32.3	28.7	57.5	52.6	48.5	0.07	0.05	0.04	-3.1	-3.2	-3.3
Minneapolis-St. Paul	21.0	23.8	29.4	36.7	41.1	50.0	0.03	0.04	0.05	-3.6	-3.5	-3.3
New York	23.6	19.9	16.3	36.5	29.5	25.0	0.02	0.02	0.01	-4.4	-4.6	-4.7
Philadelphia	28.2	21.9	19.1	40.2	33.4	28.3	0.03	0.02	0.02	-4.0	-4.2	-4.4
Portland	43.0	44.1	38.9	69.5	70.9	65.8	0.07	0.08	0.07	-2.8	-2.8	-2.9
Seattle	29.3	27.4	28.7	50.2	46.5	47.3	0.05	0.05	0.05	-3.2	-3.2	-3.2
St. Louis	29.3	23.3	16.3	43.4	36.9	34.6	0.04	0.03	0.03	-3.6	-1.9	-3.7
San Francisco-Oakland	22.6	20.7	20.9	33.2	31.7	31.4	0.03	0.03	0.03	-4.0	-4.0	-4.0
Scranton	73.7	73.0	69.5	92.8	91.6	92.9	0.24	0.23	0.18	-1.9	-1.9	-2.0
Washington	33.5	30.7	27.9	50.1	47.8	45.5	0.05	0.04	0.04	-3.3	-3.4	-3.4

Table D-2
Concentration Measures: FTE Personnel

SMSA	Four-Hospital Concentration Ratio (%)			Eight-Hospital Concentration Ratio (%)			Herfindahl Index			Entropy Index		
	1969	1972	1975	1969	1972	1975	1969	1972	1975	1969	1972	1975
Atlanta	56.3	42.1	39.4	80.2	64.5	59.5	0.11	0.08	0.07	-2.6	-2.9	-3.1
Baltimore	32.3	29.0	29.2	49.7	45.5	45.4	0.05	0.05	0.04	-3.3	-3.4	-3.4
Boston	25.9	22.7	23.5	35.8	33.4	35.6	0.30	0.25	0.03	-4.1	-4.2	-4.1
Buffalo	37.8	36.4	35.7	62.8	61.3	59.2	0.06	0.06	0.06	-2.9	-2.9	-3.0
Chattanooga	72.4	75.9	76.3	87.3	91.4	92.0	0.21	0.22	0.21	-2.0	-2.0	-2.0
Chicago	18.8	18.0	18.2	28.2	27.6	27.2	0.02	0.02	0.02	-4.4	-4.4	-4.4
Cincinnati	45.4	44.9	42.9	68.2	68.0	66.6	0.07	0.07	0.07	-2.8	-3.0	-2.9
Cleveland	32.6	32.8	35.5	50.6	50.0	51.4	0.05	0.05	0.05	-3.3	-3.4	-3.3
Dallas	39.1	37.4	35.2	59.0	57.4	55.7	0.06	0.05	0.05	-3.3	-3.4	-3.5
Denver	34.0	33.2	32.3	57.6	58.1	56.7	0.06	0.06	0.05	-3.0	-3.1	-3.1
Detroit	20.5	22.3	21.4	34.0	35.3	33.9	0.03	0.03	0.03	-3.9	-4.0	-4.0
Houston	48.5	41.9	38.8	67.1	64.2	61.5	0.08	0.06	0.06	-3.0	-3.2	-3.3
Los Angeles-Long Beach	13.3	21.9	24.3	22.7	30.5	34.0	0.01	0.02	0.03	-4.6	-4.4	-4.4
Memphis	83.9	83.1	78.7	94.7	95.3	90.8	0.20	0.26	0.19	-1.9	-1.7	-2.0
Miami	53.0	45.8	42.7	74.0	62.7	58.2	0.12	0.09	0.08	-2.6	-2.9	-3.0
Milwaukee	34.1	35.0	34.0	54.9	54.0	53.4	0.05	0.06	0.05	-3.1	-3.1	-3.2
Minneapolis-St. Paul	28.3	30.7	34.5	43.7	49.3	57.7	0.04	0.05	0.06	-3.5	-3.4	-3.1
New York	13.0	13.2	14.5	22.1	23.2	25.0	0.13	0.01	0.02	-4.7	-4.6	-4.5
Philadelphia	17.9	15.4	13.8	31.5	28.6	24.6	0.02	0.02	0.02	-4.2	-4.3	-4.4
Portland	47.1	47.5	48.9	72.8	73.6	74.6	0.08	0.08	0.09	-2.7	-2.7	-2.7
Seattle	38.3	36.8	37.0	59.0	59.3	60.3	0.06	0.06	0.06	-3.1	-3.1	-3.1
St. Louis	25.9	25.3	25.0	39.6	39.2	38.4	0.03	0.03	0.03	-3.6	-3.6	-3.6
San Francisco-Oakland	20.3	22.2	20.8	32.2	34.1	34.3	0.02	0.03	0.03	-4.0	-3.9	-3.8
Scranton	66.3	69.6	69.5	91.0	92.6	93.5	0.14	0.15	0.15	-2.2	-2.1	-2.1
Washington	30.4	29.5	29.7	51.3	48.4	49.7	0.05	0.04	0.04	-3.3	-3.4	-3.3

Appendix E
Reference Industries
for Census Analysis

Table E-1 presents the industries selected as reference industries for the analysis of U.S. census data in chapter 4. This list is a result of an attempt to match the three-digit industry code used by the Census Bureau with the four-digit SIC code used by Alexander (1974). In matching, we have taken a conservative course— that is, when the three-digit code includes industries not included in its four-digit counterpart, the three-digit code and associated observations from the Public Use Samples have been excluded from our analysis. The lists for 1960 and 1970 differ somewhat. We felt that some of the 1970 codes, not listed in 1960, are appropriate for our analysis; and to exclude industry categories where exact correspondence between the two years is not possible would restrict our sample unduly.

Table E-1
Industries Included in Reference Groups, 1960 and 1970

Industry	Census Code
Manorial Reference Group (1960)	
Miscellaneous chemicals and allied products	346
Synthetic fibers	349
Petroleum refining	377
Rubber products	379
Blast furnaces, steel works, rolling and finishing mills	139
Miscellaneous machinery (except electrical)	176
Motor vehicles and motor vehicle equipment	219
Aircraft and parts	227
Water transportation	419
Air transportation	427
Telephone (wire and radio)	448
Electric light and power	467
Gas and steam supply systems	469
Electric-gas utilities	468
Guild Reference Group (1960)	
Crude petroleum and natural gas extractions	049
Construction	066
Printing, publishing, and allied industries (except newspapers)	339
Radio broadcasting and television	447
Gasoline service stations	648
Apparel and accessories stores (except shoe stores)	657
Eating and drinking places	669
Hotels and lodging places	776
Laundering, cleaning, and other garment services	779
Barber and beauty shops	786
Engineering and architectural services	888

Table E-1 *(continued)*

Industry	Census Code
Unstructured Reference Group (1960)	
Bakery products	287
Sawmills, planing mills, and mill work	108
Pulp, paper, and paperboard mills	328
Paints, varnishes, and related products	359
Footwear (except rubber)	389
Fabricated structural metal products	158
Motor vehicles and equipment (wholesale trade)	507
Food and related products (wholesale trade)	527
Petroleum products (wholesale trade)	558
Hardware and farm equipment stores	533
General merchandise retailing	626
Food stores (except dairy products)	636
Shoe stores	658
Furniture and home furnishing stores	667
Manorial Reference Group (1970)	
Blast furnaces, steel works, rolling and finishing mills	139
Engines and turbines	177
Household appliances	199
Motor vehicles and motor vehicles equipment	219
Aircraft and parts	227
Industrial chemicals	347
Synthetic fibers	349
Petroleum refining	377
Rubber products	379
Air transportation	427
Telephone (wire and radio)	448
Electric light and power	467
Electric-gas utilities	468
Gas and steam supply systems	469
Guild Reference Group (1970)	
Crude petroleum and natural gas extractions	049
General building contractors	067
General contractors (except building)	068
Special trade contractors	069
Pulp, paper, and paperboard mills	328
Printing, publishing, and allied industries (except newspapers)	339
Water transportation	419
Radio broadcasting and television	447
Scrap and waste materials	559
Motor vehicle dealers	639
Gasoline service stations	648
Apparel and accessories stores (except shoe stores)	657
Eating and drinking places	669
Credit agencies	708
Hotels and motels	777
Laundering, cleaning, and other garment services	779
Barber shops	788
Engineering and architectural services	888
Unstructured Reference Group (1970)	
Sawmills, planing mills, and mill work	108

Table E-1 *(continued)*

Industry	Census Code
Fabricated structural metal products	158
Bakery products	287
Paperboard containers and boxes	337
Paints, varnishes, and related products	359
Footwear (except rubber)	389
Motor vehicles and equipment (wholesale trade)	507
Food and related products (wholesale trade)	527
Petroleum products (wholesale trade)	558
Lumber and building material retailing	607
Hardware and farm equipment stores	608
Miscellaneous general merchandise stores	627
Grocery stores	628
Retail bakeries	637
Tire, battery, and accessory stores	647
Shoe stores	658
Furniture and home furnishing stores	667
Drug stores	677
Business management and consulting services	738
Automobile repair and related services	757

Appendix F
Earnings Regressions
Based on Census Data

Tables F-1 and F-2 present regressions with the natural logarithm of annual earnings as the dependent variable. In contrast to hourly wages, the dependent variables in micro regressions presented in chapter 4, annual earnings, reflect both the wage rate per hour and the number of hours worked per year (estimated by multiplying the number of work hours in the reference 1960 or 1970 week, by the number of weeks worked in the previous year—1959 or 1969). We prefer the estimates in tables 4-4 and 4-5 for purposes of our analysis because the hourly wage is a more direct measure of compensation per unit of effort.

In tables F-1 and F-2, insignificant parameter estimates are the exception rather than the rule. For this reason, and to avoid needless clutter, we have not identified estimates statistically significant at conventional levels. The vast majority of parameter estimates are plausible. The interested reader may want to use the estimated earnings regressions for purposes of comparing earnings determinants in the four industry groups. Tests for regression coefficient homogeneity indicate all industry group regressions are statistically significantly different from one another.

Table F-1
Earnings Regressions, 1960

Variable	Males				Females			
	HOSP	MNOR	GULD	UNST	HOSP	MNOR	GULD	UNST
WKCC	-0.036 (0.039)	-0.232 (0.008)	-0.253 (0.013)	0.242 (0.015)	0.133 (0.024)	0.133 (0.016)	0.727 (0.022)	0.714 (0.022)
RESIDMT	0.036 (0.055)	0.616 (0.013)	0.141 (0.018)	0.176 (0.021)	0.152 (0.036)	0.131 (0.029)	0.150 (0.036)	0.681 (0.034)
URB	0.017 (0.057)	0.485 (0.015)	0.798 (0.019)	0.146 (0.021)	0.185 (0.035)	0.865 (0.031)	0.792 (0.036)	0.385 (0.035)
RACEN	-0.110 (0.060)	-0.264 (0.029)	-0.284 (0.034)	-0.232 (0.048)	-0.545 (0.046)	-0.182 (0.063)	-0.109 (0.049)	-0.134 (0.065)
SPANAME	-0.791 (0.074)	0.190 (0.020)	-0.149 (0.022)	-0.381 (0.033)	0.778 (0.041)	-0.187 (0.034)	0.314 (0.035)	0.148 (0.040)
EXPER	0.352 (0.0046)	0.357 (0.0012)	0.372 (0.0016)	0.461 (0.0018)	0.267 (0.003)	0.284 (0.002)	0.232 (0.0026)	0.192 (0.0028)
EXPSQ	-0.556 (0.00009)	-0.508 (0.00002)	-0.625 (0.00003)	-0.760 (0.00004)	-0.454 (0.00006)	-0.465 (0.00004)	-0.419 (0.00005)	-0.384 (0.00006)
NMARR	-0.100 (0.044)	-0.140 (0.014)	-0.233 (0.017)	-0.217 (0.022)	0.147 (0.027)	0.866 (0.018)	0.245 (0.026)	0.251 (0.029)
UMARR	-0.118 (0.046)	-0.756 (0.014)	-0.132 (0.018)	-0.148 (0.022)	0.602 (0.025)	0.390 (0.019)	0.913 (0.020)	0.995 (0.021)
FR1	0.111 (0.046)	0.313 (0.017)	-0.161 (0.025)	0.310 (0.032)	0.685 (0.040)	-0.910 (0.036)	-0.304 (0.038)	-0.174 (0.040)
FR2	-0.254 (0.076)	-0.465 (0.019)	-0.688 (0.023)	-0.205 (0.031)	-0.147 (0.062)	-0.110 (0.052)	-0.358 (0.043)	0.146 (0.052)
BC	0.975 (0.072)	-0.144 (0.033)	-0.119 (0.038)	-0.170 (0.054)	-0.778 (0.056)	-0.102 (0.083)	-0.615 (0.057)	-0.364 (0.089)

EDUC	-0.153 (0.022)	-0.158 (0.0061)	-0.352 (0.0069)	-0.120 (0.0091)	-0.322 (0.019)	-0.128 (0.017)	-0.311 (0.015)	-0.334 (0.020)
EDUCSQ	0.318 (0.0010)	0.330 (0.00029)	0.267 (0.00035)	0.293 (0.00045)	0.236 (0.00082)	0.234 (0.00077)	0.400 (0.00075)	0.283 (0.00097)
RESAG01	-0.122 (0.055)	-0.358 (0.014)	0.895 (0.018)	-0.666 (0.025)	-0.757 (0.033)	-0.660 (0.027)	-0.761 (0.032)	-0.168 (0.040)
CLT2	-0.499 (0.085)	0.135 (0.020)	0.443 (0.026)	0.172 (0.033)	-0.984 (0.081)	-0.457 (0.098)	-0.133 (0.086)	-0.268 (0.151)
CLT6	-0.812 (0.063)	0.273 (0.012)	0.258 (0.017)	0.210 (0.020)	-0.107 (0.050)	-0.637 (0.044)	0.102 (0.048)	-0.179 (0.058)
CLT16	0.567 (0.026)	0.134 (0.0058)	0.188 (0.0077)	-0.227 (0.0094)	-0.241 (0.022)	-0.401 (0.019)	-0.718 (0.018)	-0.116 (0.023)
CLT19	0.111 (0.056)	0.193 (0.010)	0.426 (0.015)	-0.136 (0.016)	-0.212 (0.034)	-0.110 (0.025)	-0.265 (0.027)	-0.104 (0.028)
NOREAST	-0.927 (0.076)	-0.161 (0.018)	-0.177 (0.027)	-0.189 (0.028)	-0.144 (0.047)	-0.198 (0.034)	-0.147 (0.046)	-0.269 (0.042)
MA	-0.324 (0.058)	-0.861 (0.013)	-0.923 (0.018)	-0.114 (0.022)	-0.103 (0.037)	-0.803 (0.026)	-0.208 (0.032)	-0.120 (0.033)
ENC	0.179 (0.063)	0.309 (0.013)	0.183 (0.020)	0.454 (0.022)	-0.589 (0.037)	-0.129 (0.026)	0.400 (0.032)	-0.194 (0.033)
WNC	0.235 (0.077)	-0.172 (0.019)	-0.881 (0.025)	-0.107 (0.028)	-0.177 (0.043)	-0.465 (0.034)	-0.465 (0.039)	-0.123 (0.039)
SA	-0.910 (0.075)	0.631 (0.019)	-0.104 (0.023)	-0.910 (0.027)	-0.291 (0.045)	0.950 (0.034)	0.560 (0.041)	-0.531 (0.041)
ESC	-0.112 (0.094)	0.847 (0.023)	-0.155 (0.029)	-0.126 (0.031)	-0.829 (0.057)	0.226 (0.044)	0.218 (0.054)	-0.778 (0.049)
WSC	-0.391 (0.077)	0.666 (0.018)	-0.114 (0.022)	-0.865 (0.027)	-0.137 (0.046)	-0.497 (0.033)	0.377 (0.038)	-0.683 (0.041)
MT	-0.665 (0.111)	0.671 (0.030)	0.487 (0.030)	0.841 (0.041)	-0.509 (0.058)	0.556 (0.051)	0.674 (0.050)	-0.282 (0.062)

Table F-1 *(continued)*

	Males				Females			
Variable	*HOSP*	*MNOR*	*GULD*	*UNST*	*HOSP*	*MNOR*	*GULD*	*UNST*
CONSTANT	7.564	7.876	7.695	7.635	7.306	7.65	7.16	7.62
	$R^2 = 0.25$ $F(27,734)$ $= 8.86$	$R^2 = 0.24$ $F(27,115)$ $= 136.5$	$R^2 = 0.21$ $F(27,102)$ $= 100.89$	$R^2 = 0.26$ $F(27,575)$ $= 74.27$	$R^2 = 0.13$ $F(27,277)$ $= 15.44$	$R^2 = 0.16$ $F(27,3499)$ $= 24.99$	$R^2 = 0.11$ $F(27,4728)$ $= 22.64$	$R^2 = 0.10$ $F(27,3782)$ $= 15.19$

Note: Figures in parentheses are standard errors.

Table F-2
Earnings Regressions, 1970

Variable	Males				Females			
	HOSP	MNOR	GULD	UNST	HOSP	MNOR	GULD	UNST
RESIDMT	0.078 (0.080)	-0.029 (0.035)	-0.00073 (0.029)	0.056 (0.039)	0.144 (0.045)	0.011 (0.062)	0.104 (0.051)	0.083 (0.057)
URB	-0.003 (0.091)	0.030 (0.043)	0.028 (0.035)	0.068 (0.047)	0.159 (0.052)	-0.056 (0.072)	-0.114 (0.062)	0.123 (0.067)
RACEN	0.030 (0.102)	-0.211 (0.054)	-0.171 (0.062)	0.064 (0.087)	-0.032 (0.068)	-0.155 (0.082)	-0.078 (0.092)	-0.055 (0.194)
SPANAME	-0.078 (0.141)	-0.093 (0.070)	-0.206 (0.061)	-0.088 (0.078)	-0.175 (0.100)	-0.040 (0.133)	0.105 (0.098)	0.115 (0.133)
EXPER	0.055 (0.0075)	0.048 (0.0035)	0.056 (0.0033)	0.053 (0.0044)	0.035 (0.0047)	0.036 (0.0052)	0.039 (0.0050)	0.036 (0.0061)
EXPSQ	-0.00095 (0.00015)	-0.00084 (0.00007)	-0.0011 (0.00007)	-0.00095 (0.00009)	-0.00060 (0.00010)	-0.00064 (0.00012)	-0.00074 (0.00011)	-0.00071 (0.00013)
NMARR	-0.336 (0.074)	-0.252 (0.033)	-0.386 (0.033)	-0.417 (0.045)	0.081 (0.043)	0.096 (0.042)	0.044 (0.051)	0.199 (0.059)
UMARR	-0.205 (0.086)	-0.041 (0.034)	-0.197 (0.034)	-0.180 (0.048)	0.078 (0.037)	0.123 (0.047)	0.123 (0.043)	0.180 (0.055)
FR1	0.023 (0.255)	-0.163 (0.138)	0.072 (0.106)	-0.062 (0.161)	0.218 (0.168)	0.166 (0.206)	0.169 (0.227)	0.436 (0.325)
FR2	-0.122 (0.236)	-0.339 (0.126)	0.059 (0.098)	-0.041 (0.127)	0.039 (0.153)	0.209 (0.234)	-0.118 (0.207)	0.249 (0.255)
BC	-0.186 (0.125)	0.107 (0.069)	-0.038 (0.073)	-0.189 (0.105)	-0.042 (0.078)	-0.067 (0.111)	0.047 (0.110)	0.107 (0.229)
EDUC	-0.062 (0.042)	-0.065 (0.023)	-0.054 (0.019)	0.028 (0.027)	-0.019 (0.030)	-0.024 (0.047)	-0.086 (0.040)	-0.037 (0.062)

Table F-2 *(continued)*

Variable	Males				Females			
	HOSP	MNOR	GULD	UNST	HOSP	MNOR	GULD	UNST
EDUCSQ	0.0057 (0.0018)	0.0049 (0.0010)	0.0047 (0.00087)	0.00035 (0.0012)	0.0033 (0.0013)	0.0021 (0.0021)	0.0065 (0.0019)	0.0030 (0.0029)
ACTAG01	0.275 (0.099)	0.106 (0.041)	0.145 (0.047)	0.124 (0.061)	-0.027 (0.061)	0.096 (0.084)	0.225 (0.104)	0.406 (0.123)
FR3	0.391 (0.256)	0.303 (0.132)	-0.145 (0.104)	0.065 (0.149)	-0.079 (0.165)	-0.178 (0.216)	-0.264 (0.223)	-0.200 (0.311)
P80	-0.041 (0.054)	-0.058 (0.023)	-0.115 (0.024)	-0.102 (0.033)	-0.124 (0.030)	-0.074 (0.038)	-0.180 (0.041)	-0.088 (0.051)
DISLIM1	-0.120 (0.127)	-0.200 (0.069)	-0.145 (0.069)	0.118 (0.113)	-0.190 (0.108)	-0.064 (0.154)	-0.255 (0.124)	0.082 (0.158)
DISLIM2	-0.092 (0.102)	-0.113 (0.045)	-0.157 (0.043)	-0.151 (0.057)	0.015 (0.094)	-0.112 (0.136)	-0.123 (0.095)	-0.173 (0.143)
RESAG01	0.117 (0.097)	0.072 (0.042)	0.051 (0.042)	0.068 (0.058)	0.023 (0.051)	-0.094 (0.071)	0.141 (0.064)	0.058 (0.088)
INDAG01	-0.081 (0.078)	-0.151 (0.032)	-0.170 (0.031)	-0.164 (0.040)	-0.144 (0.049)	-0.227 (0.049)	-0.146 (0.050)	-0.190 (0.059)
OCCAG01	-0.211 (0.078)	-0.032 (0.029)	-0.0068 (0.030)	-0.080 (0.039)	-0.122 (0.049)	-0.055 (0.047)	-0.157 (0.048)	-0.193 (0.058)
CLT2	0.060 (0.091)	0.060 (0.033)	0.035 (0.036)	0.077 (0.054)	-0.092 (0.068)	-0.030 (0.087)	-0.156 (0.077)	-0.025 (0.118)
CLT6	0.058 (0.054)	0.059 (0.024)	0.047 (0.024)	0.048 (0.034)	-0.065 (0.037)	0.105 (0.045)	-0.140 (0.043)	0.056 (0.054)
CLT16	-0.029 (0.029)	-0.0060 (0.012)	-0.011 (0.011)	-0.020 (0.014)	-0.037 (0.015)	-0.047 (0.018)	-0.048 (0.018)	-0.074 (0.022)
CLT19	-0.155 (0.057)	-0.027 (0.024)	-0.072 (0.022)	-0.106 (0.027)	-0.018 (0.030)	-0.078 (0.035)	-0.188 (0.033)	-0.227 (0.042)

Table F-2 *(continued)*

NOREAST	-0.087 (0.110)	-0.184 (0.055)	0.022 (0.051)	-0.117 (0.068)	-0.127 (0.067)	-0.159 (0.081)	0.035 (0.086)	-0.311 (0.094)
MA	-0.080 (0.092)	-0.073 (0.040)	0.015 (0.038)	-0.053 (0.051)	-0.067 (0.053)	-0.098 (0.061)	0.114 (0.062)	-0.109 (0.079)
ENC	0.018 (0.096)	0.051 (0.036)	0.110 (0.039)	0.131 (0.051)	-0.070 (0.054)	0.022 (0.055)	0.120 (0.059)	-0.086 (0.075)
WNC	-0.078 (0.118)	-0.035 (0.055)	0.015 (0.050)	-0.079 (0.061)	-0.148 (0.063)	-0.039 (0.081)	0.019 (0.075)	-0.137 (0.093)
SA	0.082 (0.108)	0.013 (0.047)	0.0025 (0.040)	-0.064 (0.053)	0.00073 (0.060)	0.124 (0.069)	0.212 (0.065)	-0.015 (0.087)
ESC	0.056 (0.120)	-0.081 (0.055)	-0.066 (0.052)	-0.217 (0.068)	-0.020 (0.077)	0.040 (0.090)	0.223 (0.086)	-0.122 (0.100)
WSC	0.061 (0.106)	0.087 (0.050)	-0.0072 (0.044)	-0.054 (0.060)	-0.071 (0.066)	-0.024 (0.070)	0.181 (0.072)	-0.021 (0.089)
MT	0.026 (0.182)	-0.136 (0.073)	-0.022 (0.062)	-0.018 (0.081)	-0.261 (0.091)	-0.030 (0.124)	0.243 (0.100)	-0.010 (0.125)
CONSTANT	7.714	8.397	8.122	7.798	7.601	8.011	7.532	7.476
	$R^2 = 0.55$ $F(33,306)$ $= 11.43$	$R^2 = 0.41$ $F(33,1593)$ $= 33.71$	$R^2 = 0.42$ $F(33,2715)$ $= 60.55$	$R^2 = 0.50$ $F(33,1514)$ $= 46.66$	$R^2 = 0.26$ $F(33,1280)$ $= 13.50$	$R^2 = 0.29$ $F(33,861)$ $= 10.87$	$R^2 = 0.22$ $F(33,1639)$ $= 14.12$	$R^2 = 0.26$ $F(33,876)$ $= 9.24$

Note: Figures in parentheses are standard errors.

Appendix G
Noncensus Data
Sources for the State
Regressions in
Chapter 4

The dependent variables in chapter 4 come from the Public Use Tapes of the 1960 and 1970 U.S. censuses of population; these data are described in chapter 4. Explanatory variables in the state regressions come from these sources. **REIM**: See appendix B. **INS1** and **INS2**: Variables INS1 and INS2 are estimates of depth of total private health insurance and private hospital insurance, respectively. As described more fully in Sloan and Steinwald (forthcoming, 1980), INS1 and INS2 are derived from a three-stage process. As indicated in the text, the principal data source for INS variables is verified premium data from a national household survey of health utilization and expenditures conducted in 1971 by the University of Chicago's Center for Health Administration Studies.

In the first stage, the hospital's premium is the dependent variable and explanatory variables represent (1) the benefit structure of the household's insurance policy and (2) proxies for variations in insurer profit and administrative expense (loading). Regression coefficients on the benefit structure variables represent the premium cost associated with adding or subtracting a specific benefit. Setting the profit-administrative cost variables at their mean values, indexes of depth of total and hospital coverage are calculated for each household in the sample from binary benefit structure variables and their associated coefficients. The hospital depth of coverage index is based on variables and associated coefficients most closely related to hospital services. In a second stage, demand for coverage equations are estimated with the household as the observational unit with such independent variables as income and education. Third, parameter estimates from these regressions are combined with state data on the explanatory variables to generate state INS1 and INS2 series for 1970. **MCAID**: State-local expenditures on medical assistance per capita population come from the *Statistical Abstract of the United States (SA)*. Data are for 1969. Like all monetarily expressed variables, MCAID has been deflated by a state price index expressed in 1960 dollars. See appendix A for a discussion of our price indexes. **INC**: Personal per capita income in the state for 1960 and 1970 in real 1960 dollars. Data sources are *SA*s. **MD**: Physicians per 1,000 population. Unpublished data from the American Medical Association for 1960. American Medical Association, *Distribution of Physicians* for 1970. **DENS**: Population per square mile in 1960 and 1970. Data sources are *SA*s. **LIM**: Percent of persons by state with an activity limitation due to chronic conditions,

July 1962 to July 1964. From U.S. National Center for Health Statistics, *Synthetic State Estimates of Disability* (PHS Publication no. 1759), p. 4. **HLTH**: Percent of persons by state falling into four mutually exclusive disability groups (not limited in activity; not limited in major activity but otherwise limited; limited in amount or kind or major activity performed; and unable to carry on major activity). These percentages are weighted by the number of hospital days per annum of persons in each of the four activity limitation categories. Sources: U.S. National Center for Health Statistics (1977), table 1; and U.S. National Center for Health Statistics (1976), table 7. **MW**: Manufacturing wage for 1959 and 1960 in 1960 dollars. Sources are *SA*s. **UN**: State unemployment rate. In 1960, we took state unemployment rates from the U.S. census of population. These are estimates of the proportion of the labor force looking for work as of April 1960. For the 1970 analysis, we used state unemployment rates from *SA* for 1969. **CBARG, CREQ,** and **STR**: 1970 American Hospital Association annual hospital survey, taken from public use tape. See text and/or appendix I for definitions.

Appendix H
Data Sources and
Variable Construction
for the Regression
Analysis in Chapter 5

The dependent variable is the mean annual earnings of hospital employees other than physicians, RNs, LPNs, and trainees, deflated by our area price index. The data source is annual surveys of hospitals conducted by the American Hospital Association. Explanatory variables are defined in table H-1.

Table H-1
Explanatory Variables

Variable Name	Definition	Source
INC	Per-capita income, by county, deflated by area price index	Area Resource File (1970 data), Sales Management, Inc. (1975-1976)[a]
INS	Predicted total insurance coverage index, deflated, based on 1970 estimates of insurance premium determinants—see appendix G and Sloan and Steinwald (1979)	CHAS-NORC household survey, 1970 various sources for demographic data, 1970-1975
DENS	Population per square mile, by county	American Medical Association, *Distribution of Physicians*, 1971-1976
UNEMP	Unemployment rate, by SMSA and rural areas by state	U.S. Department of Labor, *Handbook of Labor Statistics*, various years
POPMD	Population per nonhospital, patient care MD, by county	American Medical Association, *Distribution of Physicians*, 1971-1976
POPBD	Population per other hospital bed, by county (total county beds minus number of beds in the hospital)	American Medical Association, *Distribution of Physicians*, 1971-1976
GPPROP	Proportion of patient care MDs in general practice by county	American Medical Association, *Distribution of Physicians*, 1971-1976
MCAID	Proportion of population that is under 65 and eligible for Medicaid, by state	DHEW, National Center for Social Statistics *Bulletins*, 1970-1975
MCARE	Proportion of population age 65 or over, by county	Area Resource File (1970 data), Sales Management, Inc. (1975-1976)[a]
GOVT	1 for nonfederal, government hospitals; 0 otherwise	AHA annual surveys
PROP	1 for proprietary hospitals; 0 otherwise	AHA annual surveys

Table H-1 *(continued)*

Variable Name	*Definition*	*Source*
MEDSCH	1 for hospitals with medical school affiliation; 0 otherwise	AHA annual surveys
NURSCH	1 for hospitals with a professional nursing school; 0 otherwise	AHA annual surveys
SIZE1	1 if beds < 100; 0 otherwise	AHA annual surveys
SIZE2	1 if 100 ≤ beds < 250; 0 otherwise	AHA annual surveys
SIZE3	1 if 250 ≤ beds < 400; 0 otherwise	AHA annual surveys
NCON1	1 for noncomprehensive certificate-of-need program in effect for two years or less, by state; 0 otherwise	Lewin (1975); Erman (1976); Curran (1974)
NCON2	1 for noncomprehensive certificate-of-need program in effect for more than two years, by state; 0 otherwise	Lewin (1975); Erman (1976); Curran (1974)
CCON1	1 for comprehensive certificate-of-need program in effect for two years or less, by state; 0 otherwise	Lewin (1975); Erman (1976); Curran (1974)
CCON2	1 for comprehensive certificate-of-need program in effect for more than two years, by state; 0 otherwise	Lewin (1975); Erman (1976); Curran (1974)
PRECON	1 for the year prior to a certificate-of-need program taking effect, by state; 0 otherwise	Lewin (1975); Erman (1976); Curran (1974)
S1122	Proportion of population served by hospitals subject to PL 92-603, section 1122, review of capital expansion, by county	Erman (1976)[b]
BCPAA	Proportion of population served by hospitals subject to a Blue Cross requirement of local planning agency approval for reimbursement of expenses related to capital expansion, by Blue Cross plan area	AHA (1972, 1977)[b]
COSTB	Proportion of population covered by cost-based hospital reimbursement programs under Blue Cross, Medicare, and Medicaid, by insurer catchment area	AHA (1972, 1977)[b]
FPR	Proportion of population covered by formula-based prospective hospital reimbursement programs, by insurer catchment area	Lewin (1975); Laudicina (1976)[b]
BPR	Proportion of population covered by budget-based prospective hospital reimbursement programs, by insurer catchment area	Lewin (1975); Laudicina (1976)[b]
UR	Proportion of population covered by Blue Cross and Medicaid programs requiring utilization review, by state, 1974	Lewin (1975)[b]

Table H-1 *(continued)*

Variable Name	Definition	Source
ESP	Proportion of months in a year that the Economic Stabilization Program was in effect	
CBARG	See appendix I	
CBREQ	See appendix I	
STR	See appendix I	

aEstimates for the remaining years were obtained by interpolation. This was necessary since Sales Management's income and age distribution series for the early 1970s are not directly comparable to its estimates for later years. Earlier estimates are based on the 1960 census; later ones use the 1970 census. The income and age data from the Health Resource Administration's (DHEW) Area Resource File are projections based on the 1970 census.

bAdditional data sources are required to estimate population proportions covered by each reimbursement program. See appendix J.

Appendix I
Unionization Measures for Chapter 5 Based on American Hospital Association Surveys

Variable Name. CBREQ, CBARG, STR.

Description. These variables encompass hospital-specific union activities affecting some fraction of the hospital's employees (see chapters 3 and 4 for definitions). Data for construction of CBREQ and CBARG were available for 1970, 1973, and 1975 from unpublished American Hospital Association (AHA) Surveys. Data for construction of STR were available only for 1970 and 1973 from the AHA. In 1970 and 1973, the AHA question on CBREQ asked whether the hospital had, "... received a request for recognition as a collective bargaining agent ... ," and in 1975 that "... unions or other employee organizations had conducted any organizing activities for the purpose of collective bargaining among employees of the hospital ...." These two questions have been treated as equivalent. CBARG in each year indicates the presence of a signed collective bargaining agreement. STR indicates that a strike or other kind of work stoppage had occurred during the previous twelve months.

Methodology. CBREQ, CBARG, and STR have been constructed as dummy variables. To construct value for all years included in our analysis, it was necessary to estimate values for these variables for the years for which no data were available. Three assumptions were made: (1) If the data indicated the absence of a unionization "event" for two years, it was assumed to be absent in all intervening years; (2) once one of the unionization "events" took place, it was assumed that its impact would be realized throughout the remainder of the period of the study; and (3) for hospitals indicating that they had a signed collective bargaining agreement in a given year, it was assumed that it was equally likely that the agreement was signed in any prior year following a year when no such agreement was indicated. Potential values of the three variables and means for the sample are shown in table I-1.

Table I-1
Potential Values of Unionization Variables

Variable	Year					
	1970	1971	1972	1973	1974	1975
CBREQ	0	0	0	0	0	0
	0	0	0	0	0	1
	0	0	0	1	1	1
	1	1	1	1	1	1
CBARG	0	0	0	0	0	0
	0	0	0	0	.5	1
	0	.33	.67	1	1	1
	1	1	1	1	1	1
STR	0	0	0	0	0	0
	0	0	0	1	1	1
	1	1	1	1	1	1

Note: The table shows all possible values of each variable for any given hospital for each of the six years. As defined, for any sample hospital, the value of a unionization variable in a given year must be equal to or greater than the value in the preceding year. Sample means of CBREQ, CBARG, and STR across all years are .25, .24, and .05, respectively.

Appendix J
Estimates of
Proportions of Persons
Covered by Specific
Reimbursement
Programs for the
Analysis in Chapter 5

We assume that the effectiveness of all regulatory programs varies directly with the proportion of the population covered. Thus population proportions are used in computation of the regulation variables, S1122, BCPAA, COSTB, FPR, BPR, UR.

All reimbursement variables, excluding ESP, require estimation of area population proportions covered by the different reimbursement programs. With regard to hospital reimbursement, populations are classified as falling into one or more of the following categories (units of observation of area data are also shown):

Blue Cross enrolled . . . by Blue Cross plan area.

Medicare eligible . . . by county.

Medicaid eligible . . . by state.

Commercial insurance enrolled . . . estimated from above data.

Blue Cross Association publishes annual figures on proportion of plan area population enrolled in Blue Cross plans. These data were used to construct the area Blue Cross enrollment proportion variable (BCP). The seventy-one Blue Cross plan areas (United States and Puerto Rico, as of December 31, 1975) are combinations of contiguous counties. In many cases, one Blue Cross plan serves an entire state. In other cases, two or more plans exist within a state, and in a few cases plan areas cross state lines. The value of BCP for a given hospital and year depends on the hospital's location with regard to Blue Cross plan area boundaries.

Proportions of county population age sixty-five and over (MCARE) is used as our measure of Medicare eligibility. Although some persons age sixty-five and over are not eligible for Medicare, and some people under age sixty-five are eligible, these cases are ufficiently small in magnitude to be ignored in the area proportion estimates. MCARE is measured directly for 1975 from data published by Sales Management, Inc., and for 1970, using data obtained from the Area Resource File, compiled and distributed by the Bureau of Health Manpower, DHEW. In between years' proportions were estimated via linear interpolation, a process that is subject to very slight estimation error.

Medicaid eligibility data are available by year, but only for states. Two Medicaid variables have been defined: the proportion of state population eligible for Medicaid (MCDP) and the proportion of state population under sixty-five and eligible for Medicaid (MCAID). The latter variable is employed whenever Medicare proportions are added to Medicaid proportions to avoid double counting. Because Medicaid variables are computed with state data, they are subject to some erors in variables. Moreover, when Medicaid proportions are combined with other area proportion data (for example, when MCARE and MCAID are summed to obtain county population proportions subject to Section 1122 reimbursement regulation), this implicitly assumes that the Medicaid proportion is constant across counties within the state.

The remaining proportion variable, COMP, which measures the proportion of area population with commercial hospital insurance coverage, is very crudely estimated but used in very few instances. Commercial reimbursement tends to be subject to regulation far less frequently than the Blue Cross and governmental reimbursement programs. Moreover, when commercial reimbursement is covered by a particular regulation, it is frequently true that *all* reimbursement within a state is covered, such that the area proportion can safely be estimated to be 1.0. The only cases wherein nonstatewide regulation includes commercial reimbursement are prospective reimbursement in Arizona and Connecticut. In these cases, the proportion of population with no insurance or with "other" insurance (nongovernmental, non-Blue Cross, noncommercial) was assumed to equal 0.05. The area proportion with commercial insurance was estimated as follows: COMP - .95 - BCP-MCARE-MCAID. Because this formula was used so infrequently, a more precise estimating system was deemed unnecessary.

Table J-1 provides estimates of annual means of the primary area proportion variables and the regulation variables for 1970-1975. Grand means of these variables and percentage increases from 1970-1975 are also shown.

Table J-1
Sample Means of Primary Area Population and Reimbursement Proportion Variables, 1970-1975

	Population Proportions by Payor and Year						*Grand Mean*	*Percent Increase 1970-1975*
	1970	*1971*	*1972*	*1973*	*1974*	*1975*		
BCP	.369	.373	.380	.393	.402	.408	.387	10.6
MCARE	.097	.098	.098	.101	.102	.102	.100	5.2
MCDP	.095	.098	.102	.100	.113	.117	.104	23.2
MCAID	.074	.077	.081	.082	.092	.096	.084	29.7

Table J-1 *(continued)*

	Population Proportions by Payor and Year						Grand Mean	Percent Increase 1970-1975
	1970	*1971*	*1972*	*1973*	*1974*	*1975*		
Resulting Regulation Variables Included in the Analysis in Chapter 5								
S1122	.000	.000	.000	.041	.102	.105	.041	
BCPAA	.149	.149	.150	.219	.224	.226	.186	51.7
COST	.479	.485	.489	.502	.521	.529	.501	10.4
FPR	.088	.089	.090	.092	.096	.109	.094	23.9
BPR	.029	.030	.048	.061	.086	.087	.057	200.0
UR	.351	.357	.359	.364	.380	.384	.366	9.4
ESP	.000	.250	1.000	1.000	.250	.000	.417	

Bibliography

Abt Associates, Inc., and Policy Analysis, Inc. *Analysis of Prospective Payment Systems for Upstate New York.* Final Report under contract no. HEW-OS 74-261 to the Social Security Administration, April 6, 1976.

Alchian, Armen A., and Kessel, Reuben A. "Competition, Monopoly, and the Pursuit of Pecuniary Gain." In *Aspects of Labor Economics: A Conference of the Universities-National Bureau for Economic Research Committee*, pp. 156-175. Princeton, N.J.: Princeton University Press, 1962.

Alexander, A.J. "Income, Experience, and Internal Labor Markets." *The Quarterly Journal of Economics* 88, no. 2 (February 1974).

Altman, S.H. *Present and Future Supply of Registered Nurses.* Washington, D.C.: U.S. Department of Health, Education, and Welfare, National Institutes of Health, Division of Nursing, 1971.

Altman, S.H., and Eichenholz, Joseph. "Inflation in the Health Industry—Causes and Cures." In Zubkoff, ed. *Health: A Victim or Cause of Inflation.* New York: Prodist, 1976.

Altman, S.H., and Weiner, S.L. "Regulation as Second Best." In W. Greenberg, ed. *Competition in the Health Care Sector: Past, Present and Future*, pp. 421-447. Germantown, Maryland: Aspen Systems, 1978.

American Hospital Association. "Statistical Profile of the Nation's Hospitals." In *Hospital Statistics, 1976 Edition.* Chicago: the Association, 1976.

_____. "Statistical Profile of the Nation's Hospitals." In *Hospital Statistics, 1977 Edition.* Chicago: the Association, 1978.

_____. Bureau of Fiscal Services. "Survey of Provisions of Hospital-Blue Cross Contracts at September 30, 1971." Chicago: the Association, January 1972.

_____. Division of Financial Management. "Blue Cross Contract Provisions as of June 30, 1976." Chicago: the Association, January 1977.

American Medical Association, Center for Health Services Research and Development. *Distribution of Physicians in the United States, 1970-1975.* Chicago: the Association, 1971-1976.

Baird, William. "Barriers to Collective Bargaining in Registered Nursing." *Labor Law Journal* (January 1969):42-46.

Becker, Brian. "Union Effects on Employment Stability in Low Wage Markets: Some Evidence from the Hospital Industry." Mimeograph, 1977.

Blaug, Mark. "Human Capital Theory: A Slightly Jaundiced Survey." *Journal of Economic Literature* 14, no. 3 (September 1976):827-855.

Bluestone, Barry. "The Tripartite Economy: Labor Markets and the Working Poor." *Poverty and Human Resources Abstracts* 5, no. 4 (July/August 1970):15-35.

Blumstein, J.F., and Sloan, F.A. "Health Planning and Regulation Through

Certificate of Need: An Overview." *Utah Law Review* no 1 (1978):3-38.

Bovbjerg, Randall. "Problems and Prospects for Health Planning: The Importance of Incentives, Standards, and Procedures." *Utah Law Review* no. 1 (1978):83-122.

Brown, D.G. "Expected Ability to Pay and Interindustry Wage Structure in Manufacturing." *Industrial and Labor Relations Review* 16 (October 1962):45-62.

Cain, Glen G. "The Challenge of Segmented Labor Market Theories to Orthodox Theory: A Survey." *Journal of Economic Literature* 14, no. 4 (December 1976):1215-1257.

Cotterill, Philip G., and Wadycki, Walter J. "Teenagers and the Minimum Wage in Retail Trade." *Journal of Human Resources* 11, no. 1 (Winter 1976):69-85.

Curran, W.J. "A National Survey and Analysis of State Certificate-of-Need Laws for Health Facilities." In C.C. Havighurst, ed. *Regulating Health Facilities Construction,* pp. 85-111. Washington, D.C.: American Enterprise Institute, 1974.

Davis, Karen. "Economic Theories of Behavior in Nonprofit, Private Hospitals." *Economic and Business Bulletin* 24 (Spring 1972):1-13.

_____. "Theories of Hospital Inflation: Some Empirical Evidence." *Journal of Human Resources* 8, no. 2 (Spring 1973):181-201.

Doeringer, Peter B., and Piore, Michael J. *Internal Labor Markets and Manpower Analysis.* Lexington, Mass.: Lexington Books, D.C. Heath, 1971.

Douglas, Paul H. *The Theory of Wages.* New York: Macmillan, 1934.

Dowling, W.L. "Prospective Reimbursement of Hospitals." *Inquiry* 11, no. 3 (September 1974):163-180.

Dunlop, J.T. "The Task of Contemporary Wage Theory." In G. Taylor and F. Pierson, eds. *New Concepts in Wage Determination,* pp. 117-139. New York: McGraw-Hill, 1957.

Eckstein, Otto, and Wilson, Thomas A. "The Determinants of Money Wages in American Industry." *Quarterly Journal of Economics* 76, no. 3 (August 1962):379-414.

Elnicki, Richard. "Turnover." In F. Sloan, ed. *The Geographic Distribution of Nurses and Public Policy,* pp. 117-139. Bethesda, Md.: U.S. Department of Health, Education, and Welfare, 1975.

Elnicki, Richard, and Sloan, Frank. "Normative Measures of Nurse Distribution: Evidence from the Survey of Directors of Nursing." In F. Sloan, ed. *The Geographic Distribution of Nurses and Public Policy,* pp. 81-115. Bethesda, Md.: U.S. Department of Health, Education, and Welfare, 1975.

Enthoven, Alain C. "Consumer-Choice Health Plan (First of Two Parts)." *New England Journal of Medicine* 298, no. 12 (March 23, 1978a):650-658.

_____. "Consumer-Choice Health Plan (Second of Two Parts)." *New England Journal of Medicine* 298, no. 13 (March 30, 1978b):709-720.

Erman, David. "Working Paper on Certificate of Need." Mimeograph, 1976.

Evans, Robert G. "Efficiency Incentives in Hospital Reimbursement." Ph.D. dissertation, Harvard University, 1970.

Fein, Rashi, and Bishop, Christine. *Employment Impacts of Health Policy Developments.* A Special Report of the National Commission for Manpower Policy, special report no. 11, October 1976.

Feldman, Roger D., and Scheffler, Richard M. "The Effect of Labor Unions on Hospital Employees' Wages." Mimeograph, 1977.

Feldstein, Martin S. "Econometric Studies of Health Economics." In M.D. Intriligator and D.A. Kendrick, eds. *Frontiers of Quantitative Studies, II,* pp. 377-433. Amsterdam: North Holland, 1974.

_____. *The Rising Cost of Hospital Care.* Washington: Information Resources Press, 1971.

_____. "Summary of Limiting the Rise in Hospital Costs without Regulations." Testimony before the Senate Health Subcommittee, March 15, 1979.

Feldstein, Martin, and Taylor, Amy K. "The Rapid Rise of Hospital Costs." Discussion paper no. 531, Harvard Institute of Economic Research, January 1977.

Fogel, W., and Levin, D. "Wage Determination in the Public Sector." *Industrial and Labor Relations Review* 27, no. 3 (April 1974):410-431.

Fottler, M.D. "The Union Impact on Hospital Wages." *Industrial and Labor Relations Review* 30, no. 3 (April 1977):342-355.

Fuchs, Victor R. "The Earnings of Allied Health Personnel—Are Health Workers Underpaid?" *Explorations in Economic Research* 3, no. 3 (Summer 1976):408-432.

Furst, R.W., and Dunkelberg, J.S. "Study Shows ESP Reduced Hospitals' Profitability." *Hospital Progress* (August 1978):59-63.

Galbraith, John Kenneth. *The New Industrial State.* Boston: Houghton Mifflin, 1967.

Gaus, C.R., and Hellinger, F.J. "Results of Prospective Reimbursement." *Topics in Health Care Financing* 3, no. 2 (Winter 1976):83-96.

Getz, Malcom, and Huang, Yuh-ching. "Consumer Revealed Preference for Environmental Goods." *The Review of Economics and Statistics* 60, no. 3 (August 1978):449-458.

Gibson, Robert M., and Fisher, Charles R. "National Health Expenditures, Fiscal Year 1977." *Social Security Bulletin* 41, no. 7 (July 1978):4-20.

Ginsburg, Paul B. *The Impact of the Economic Stabilization Program on Hospitals and Hospital Care.* Final Report to Department of Health, Education, and Welfare under contract HSM 110-73-467, October 15, 1976.

_____. "Impact of the Economic Stabilization Program on Hospitals: An Analysis with Aggregate Data." In M. Zubkoff, I. Raskin, and R.S. Hanft, eds. *Hospital Cost Containment,* pp. 293-323. New York: Prodist, 1978.

Gramlich, Edward. "The Impact of Minimum Wages on Other Wages, Employment and Family Incomes." *Brookings Papers on Economic Activity* 7, no. 2 (1976):409-451.

Hammermesh, David. "Market Power and Wage Inflation." *Southern Economic Journal* 34 (October 1972):204-212.

Hanoch, Giora. "Personal Earnings and Investment in Schooling." Ph.D. dissertation, University of Chicago, 1965.

Harris, Jeffrey E. "The Internal Organization of Hospitals: Some Economic Implications." *Bell Journal of Economics* 8, no. 2 (Autumn 1977):467-482.

Havighurst, Clark C. "Controlling Health Care Costs: Strengthening the Private Sector's Hand." *Journal of Health Politics, Policy and Law* 1, no. 4 (Winter 1977):471-498.

Havighurst, Clark C., and Blumstein, James F. "Coping with Quality/Cost Trade-offs in Medical Care: The Role of PSROs." *Northwestern University Law Review* 70 (March-April 1975):6-68.

Hellinger, Fred J. "The Effect of Certificate of Need Legislation on Hospital Investment." *Inquiry* 13, no. 2 (June 1976):187-193.

Hendricks, Wallace. "Regulation and Labor Earnings." *The Bell Journal of Economics* 8, no. 2 (Autumn 1977):483-496.

Hughes, Edward F.X.; Baron, David P.; Dittman, David A.; Friedman, Bernard S.; Longest, Jr., Beaufort B.; Pauly, Mark V.; and Smith, Kenneth R. *Hospital Cost Containment Programs, A Policy Analysis.* Cambridge, Mass.: Ballinger, 1978.

Hurd, Richard W. "Equilibrium Vacancies in a Labor Market Dominated by Nonprofit Firms: The 'Shortage' of Nurses." *The Review of Economics and Statistics* 55 no. 2 (May 1973):234-240.

Iowa Law Review. "Exemption of Nonprofit Hospital Employees from the National Labor Relations Act: A Violation of Equal Protection." 57 (1971-1972):412-450.

Jelinek, Richard C., and Dennis, Lyman C. *A Review and Evaluation of Nursing Productivity.* Bethesda, Md.: U.S. Department of Health, Education, and Welfare, Public Health Service, Health Resources Administration, Division of Nursing, 1976.

Katz, Arnold. "Teenage Employment Effects of State Minimum Wages." *Journal of Human Resources* 8, no. 2 (Spring 1973):250-256.

Kelly, Lucie Young. "Nursing Practice Acts." *American Journal of Nursing* 74, no. 7 (July 1974):1310-1319.

Kerr, Clark. "The Balkanization of Labor Markets." In W.W. Bakke et al., eds. *Labor Mobility and Economic Opportunity*, pp. 92-110. New York: Wiley; and Cambridge, Mass.: MIT Press, 1954.

_____ . "Labor Markets: Their Character and Consequences." *American Economic Review* 40, no. 2 (May 1950):278-291.

Kochan, Thomas A. "Correlates of State Public Employee Bargaining Laws." *Industrial Relations* 12, no. 3 (October 1973):322-337.

Kopit, W.G.; Kirll, E.J.; and Bonnie, K.F. "Hospital Decertification: Legitimate Regulation or a Taking of Private Property?" *Utah Law Review* no. 1 (1978):179-210.

Kosters, Marvin, and Welch, Finis. "The Effects of Minimum Wages on the Distribution of Changes in Aggregate Employment." *American Economic Review* 62 (June 1972):323-332.

Kumar, P. "Differentials in Wage Rates of Unskilled Labor in Canadian Manufacturing Industries." *Industrial and Labor Relations Review* 26, no. 1 (October 1972):631-645.

Landon, J.H. "The Effect of Product-Market Concentration on Wage Levels: An Intra-Industry Approach." *Industrial Labor Relations Review* 23, no. 2 (January 1970):237-247.

Landon, J.H., and Baird, R.N. "Monopsony in the Market for Public School Teachers." *American Economic Review* 61, no. 5 (December 1971):996-971.

Laudicina, S.S. *Prospective Reimbursement for Hospitals: A Guide for Policymakers.* New York: Community Service Society, October 1976.

Lee, Lung-Fei. "Unionism and Wage Rates: A Simultaneous Equations Model with Qualitative and Limited Dependent Variables." *International Economic Review* 19, no. 2 (June 1978):415-433.

Lee, Maw Lin. "A Conspicuous Production Theory of Hospital Behavior." *Southern Economic Journal* 38, no. 1 (July 1971):48-58.

Leibenstein, Harvey. "An Interpretation of the Economic Theory of Fertility: Promising Path or Blind Alley?" *Journal of Economic Literature* 12, no. 2 (June 1974):457-479.

Lewin and Associates, Inc. *An Analysis of State and Regional Health Regulation.* Final report to the Health Resources Administration under contract no. HEW-OS-73-212, February 1975.

Lewis, H.G. *Unionism and Relative Wages in the United States.* Chicago: University of Chicago Press, 1963.

Link, Charles R., and Landon, John H. "Market Structure, Nonpecuniary Factors, and Professional Salaries: Registered Nurses." *Journal of Economics and Business* 28, no. 2 (Winter 1976):151-155.

_____. "Monopsony and Union Power in the Market for Nurses." *Southern Economic Review* 41, no. 4 (April 1975):649-659.

Livernash, E. Robert. "The Internal Wage Structure." In George W. Taylor and Frank C. Pierson, eds. *New Concepts in Wage Determination,* pp. 140-172. New York: McGraw-Hill, 1957.

McClure, Walter. *Reducing Excess Hospital Capacity.* Prepared for the Bureau of Health Planning and Resources Development, Department of Health, Education, and Welfare under contract no. HRA-230-76-0086. Excelsior, Minn.: InterStudy, October 15, 1976.

McMahon, J.A., and Drake, D.F. "The American Hospital Association Perspective." In M. Zubkoff; I. Raskin; and R.S. Hanft, eds. *Hospital Cost Containment,* pp. 76-102. New York: Prodist, 1978.

Maddala, G.S. *Econometrics.* New York: McGraw-Hill, 1977.

Miller, Richard U.; Becker, Brian B.; and Krinsky, Edward B. "Union Effects on Hospital Administration: Preliminary Results from a Three-State Study." *Labor Law Journal* 28, no. 8 (August 1977):512-519.

Miller, J.D., and Shortell, S.M. "Hospital Unionization: A Study of the Trends." *Hospitals* 43 (August 1969):67-73.

Mincer, Jacob. "The Distribution of Labor Incomes: A Survey with Special Reference to the Human Capital Approach." *Journal of Economic Literature*, 8, no. 1 (March 1970):1-26.

_____. *Schooling, Experience, and Earnings*. National Bureau of Economic Research. New York: Columbia University Press, 1974.

_____. "Unemployment Effects of Minimum Wages." *Journal of Political Economy* 84, part 2 (August 1976):S87-S104.

Morley, Samuel A. *Inflation and Unemployment* 2nd ed. Hinsdale, Ill.: Dryden Press, 1979.

Nerlove, Marc. "Further Evidence on the Estimation of Dynamic Economic Relations from a Time Series of Cross Sections." *Econometrica* 39, no. 2 (March 1971):359-382.

Newhouse, Joseph P. *The Economics of Medical Care: A Policy Perspective*. Reading, Mass.: Addison-Wesley, 1978.

_____. "Toward a Theory of Nonprofit Institutions: An Economic Model of the Hospital." *American Economic Review* 60, no. 1 (March 1970):64-74.

Nickell, S.J. "Wage Structures and Quit Rates." *International Economic Review* 17, no. 1 (February 1976):191-203.

Olsen, Randall J. "Comment on the Effect of Unions on Earnings and Earnings on Unions: A Mixed Logit Approach." *International Economic Review* 19, no. 1 (February 1978):259-261.

Parsons, Donald O. "Specific Human Capital: An Application to Quit Rates and Layoff Rates." *Journal of Political Economy* 80, no. 6 (November/December 1972):1120-1143.

Pauly, Mark V., and Drake, David F. "Effect of Third-Party Methods of Reimbursement on Hospital Performance." In H.E. Klarman, ed. *Empirical Studies in Health Economics*, pp 297-314. Baltimore: Johns Hopkins Press, 1970.

Pauly, Mark, and Redisch, Michael. "The Not-for-Profit Hospital as a Physicians' Cooperative." *American Economic Review* 63, no. 1 (March 1973):87-100.

Pencavel, John H. *An Analysis of the Quit Rate in American Manufacturing Industry*. Princeton, N.J.: Industrial Relations Section, Department of Economics, Princeton University, 1970.

_____. "Wages, Specific Training and Labor Turnover in U.S. Manufacturing Industries." *International Economic Review* 13 (February 1972):53-64.

Price, James L. *The Study of Turnover*. Ames, Iowa: Iowa State University Press, 1977.

Reder, Melvin W. "The Theory of Occupational Wage Differentials." *American Economic Review* 45, no. 1 (December 1955):833-852.

Rees, Albert. *The Economics of Work and Pay.* 1st ed. New York: Harper & Row, 1973.

————. *The Economics of Work and Pay.* 2nd ed. New York: Harper & Row, 1979.

Reinhardt, Uwe E. "Comment on Sloan and Feldman, 'Competition Among Physicians." In Warren Greenberg, ed. *Competition in the Health Care Sector: Past Present, and Future,* pp. 156-190. Germantown, Md.: Aspen Systems, 1978.

Roemer, Milton I. "Bed Supply and Hospital Utilization: A Natural Experiment." *Hospitals* 35, no. 21 (November 1961):36-42.

Roemer, Milton I., and Shain, Max. *Hospital Utilization under Insurance.* Chicago: American Hospital Association, 1959.

Rosen, Sherwin. "A Wage-Based Index of Urban Quality of Life." Mimeograph, undated.

————. "Trade Union Power, Threat Effects, and the Extent of Organization." *Review of Economic Studies* 36, no. 2 (April 1969):185-196.

Rosenthal, Gerald. *The Demand for General Hospital Facilities.* Chicago: American Hospital Association, 1964.

Sales Management, Inc. *1975 Survey of Buying Power.*

————. *1976 Survey of Buying Power.*

Salkever, David S. "Competition Among Hospitals." In W. Greenberg, ed. *Competition in the Health Care Sector: Past, Present, and Future,* pp. 149-162. Germantown, Md.: Aspen Systems Corporation, 1978.

————. "Hospital Wage Inflation: Supply-Push or Demand-Pull?" *Quarterly Review of Economics and Business* 15, no. 3 (Autumn 1975):33-48.

————. "A Microeconomic Study of Hospital Cost Inflation." *Journal of Political Economy* 80, no. 6 (November/December 1972):1144-1166.

Salkever, David S., and Bice, Thomas W. "The Impact of Certificate-of-Need Controls on Hospital Investment." *Milbank Memorial Fund Quarterly* 54 (Spring 1976a):185-214.

————. *Impact of State Certificate-of-Need Laws on Health Care Costs and Utilization.* NCHSR Research Digest Series, Department of Health, Education, and Welfare, publication no. (HRA) 77-3163, 1976b.

Schmidt, Peter, and Strauss, Robert. "The Effect of Unions on Earnings and Earnings on Unions: A Mixed Logit Approach." *International Economic Review* 17, no. 1 (February 1976):204-212.

Schramm, Carl J. "The Role of Hospital Cost-Regulating Agencies in Collective Bargaining." *Labor Law Journal* (August 1977):519-525.

Schultz, T. Paul. *Estimating Labor Supply Functions for Married Women.* Santa Monica, Calif.: Rand Corporation, 1975.

Sigmond, Robert M. "How Should Blue Cross Reimburse Hospitals?" 'Costs!' " *Modern Hospital* 101, no. 1 (July 1963):91-94.

Sloan, Frank A. *Equalizing Access to Nursing Services: The Geographic Dimension.* Washington, D.C.: U.S. Government Printing Office, Department of Health, Education, and Welfare, 1978.

_____. *The Geographic Distribution of Nurses and Public Policy*. Bethesda, Md.: U.S. Department of Health, Education, and Welfare, Publication no. (HRA) 75-53, May 1975.

Sloan, Frank A., and Elnicki, Richard. "Professional Nurse Wage-Setting in Hospitals." In Richard Scheffler, ed. *Research in Health Economics*, pp. 217-254. Greenwich, Conn.: JAI Press, 1979.

Sloan, Frank A., and Feldman, Roger D. "Competition Among Physicians." In W. Greenberg, ed. *Competition in the Health Care Sector: Past, Present, and Future*, pp. 45-102. Germantown, Md.: Aspen Systems, 1978.

Sloan, Frank A., and Steinwald, Bruce. *Insurance, Regulation, and Hospital Costs*. Lexington, Mass.: Lexington Books, D.C. Heath, forthcoming, 1980.

Stafford, Frank D. "Concentration and Labor Earnings: Comment." *American Economic Review* 58, no. 1 (March 1968):79-99.

Subcommittee on Health of the Committee on Ways and Means, U.S. House of Representatives. *National Health Insurance Resource Book*. Washington, D.C.: U.S. Government Printing Office, 1976.

Taylor, Amy K. "Government Health Policy and Hospital Labor Costs: A Study of the Determinants of Hospital Wage Rates and Employment." Harvard School of Public Health, mimeograph, December 1977.

TeKolste, Elton. "How Should Blue Cross Reimburse Hospitals? 'Charges!' " *Modern Hospital* 101, no. 1 (July 1963):90, 92-94, 142.

Thaler, Richard, and Rosen, Sherwin. "The Value of Saving a Life: Evidence from the Labor Market." In Nestor E. Terleckyj, ed. *Household Production and Consumption*, pp. 265-297. New York: National Bureau of Economic Research, 1975.

Thurow, Lester C. *Generating Inequality, Mechanisms of Distribution in the U.S. Economy*. New York: Basic Books, 1975.

U.S. Department of Commerce, Bureau of the Census. *Statistical Abstract of the United States: 1977*. 98th ed. Washington, D.C.: U.S. Government Printing Office, 1977.

U.S. Department of Health, Education, and Welfare, Bureau of Health Manpower. *The Area Resource File: A Manpower Planning and Research Tool*. Data from various sources on computer tape, various years.

U.S. Department of Health, Education, and Welfare, Public Health Service. *State Estimates of Disability and Utilization of Medical Services: United States, 1969-1971*. Washington, D.C.: U.S. Government Printing Office, 1977.

U.S. Department of Health, Education, and Welfare, Bureau of Health Planning and Resources Development. *Status of Certificate-of-Need and 1122 Programs in the States, 1978*.

U.S. Department of Health, Education, and Welfare, Bureau of Health Resources Development. *The Supply of Health Manpower: 1970 Profiles and Projections for 1990*. Washington, D.C.: U.S. Government Printing Office, 1974.

U.S. Department of Labor, Bureau of Labor Statistics. *Area Wage Surveys.* 4 bulletins. Washington, D.C.: Bureau of Labor Statistics, 1967-1970.

_____. *Handbook of Labor Statistics.* Washington, D.C.: U.S. Government Printing Office, various years.

_____. *Industry Wage Survey: Hospitals, August 1975–January 1976,* bulletin 1949. Washington, D.C.: U.S. Government Printing Office, 1977.

U.S. Department of Labor, Bureau of Labor Statistics and U.S. Department of Health, Education, and Welfare, Public Health Service. "State Licensing of Health Occupations." Washington, D.C.: U.S. Government Printing Office, publication no. 1758, 1968.

U.S. Environmental Protection Agency. *Quality of Life Indicators in U.S. Metropolitan Areas: A Comprehensive Assessment.* Washington, D.C.: U.S. Government Printing Office, 1975.

U.S. Health Manpower Commission. *Report of the National Advisory Commission on Health Manpower.* vol. II. Washington, D.C.: U.S. Government Printing Office, 1967.

U.S. National Center for Health Statistics, Department of Health, Education, and Welfare. *Health Characteristics of Persons with Chronic Activity Limitation, United States–1974.* Washington, D.C.: U.S. Government Printing Office, data from National Health Survey, series 10, no. 112, DHEW publication no. (HRA) 77-1539, 1976.

Wachtel, H.M., and Betsey, C. "Employment at Low Wages." *Review of Economics and Statistics* 54, no. 2 (May 1972):121-128.

Wachter, Michael L. "Primary and Secondary Labor Markets: A Critique of the Dual Approach." *Brookings Papers on Economic Activity* 3 (1974):637-693.

Weiss, Leonard. "Concentration and Labor Earnings." *American Economic Review* 56, no. 1 (March 1966):96-117.

Weiss, R.D. "The Effect of Education on the Earnings of Blacks and Whites." *Review of Economics and Statistics* 52, no. 2 (May 1970):150-159.

Welch, Finis. "Minimum Wage Legislation in the United States." *Economic Inquiry* 12 (September 1974):285-318.

_____. "Minimum Wage Legislation in the United States: Reply." *Economic Inquiry* 15, no. 1 (January 1977):139-142.

Wennberg, John E., and Gittelsohn, Alan. "Small Area Variations in Health Care Delivery. A population-based health information system can guide planning and regulatory decisionmaking." *Science* 182 (December 1973):1102-1108.

Worthington, Paul N. "Prospective Reimbursement of Hospitals to Promote Efficiency: New Jersey." *Inquiry* 13, no. 3 (September 1976):302-308.

Yett, Donald E. *An Economic Analysis of the Nurse Shortage.* Washington, D.C.: U.S. Government Printing Office, 1970.

Index

Abt Associates, Inc., 90
Aides-orderlies, 23, 24; trends in wages of, 25
Aid to Families with Dependent Children, 28
Alexander, Arthur, 51-53, 65, 150
American Hospital Association (AHA), 12, 70, 82, 88, 114; annual hospital surveys of, 3, 6, 7, 30, 90, 91, 105, 123
Area price indexes, 138-140
Auto thefts, 32-33, 42-43

Baird, R.N., 33
Becker, Brian B., 30-31
Bice, Thomas W., 86, 95
Bishop, Christine, 54
Blue Cross, 34, 81, 89, 90, 96; Planning Agency approval variable (BCPAA), 87, 96, 126-127
Brown, D.G., 17

Capital-facilities regulation, 81, 84-87
Carter, Jimmy, 113
Census analysis, reference industries for, 150-152
Center for Health Administration Studie (CHAS), 69
Certificate-of-need (CON) laws, 81, 84-87, 95-96
Collective bargaining in hospitals, 144-146. *See also* Unionization
Compression, hospital wage-scale, 128-129
Cost-push theory of hospital wage inflation, 21-22
Cotterill, Philip G., 28
Current Population Surveys, 129

Data, 90-91
Davis, Karen, 25, 30, 74, 96; and hospital density, 33; and monopsony, 44, 133

Demand-pull theory of hospital wage inflation, 22
Doeringer, Peter, 51
Douglas, Paul, 16
Dowling, W.L., 88-89
Dunlop, J.T., 16

Earnings and employment, trends in, 3-6. *See also* Wage(s)
Earnings regressions based on census data, 153-159
Economic Stabilization Program (ESP), 7, 8, 82, 126; exemptions from, 105, 113; and revenue-cost regulation, 81, 87-88, 96
Elnicki, Richard, 29-30, 31, 42, 50
Empirical results, 97-101; overview of 35; of state cross-section analysis, 70-76; supply-side, 38-44
Empirical specification, 91-96; dependent variables and choice of labor categories for, 23-25; explanatory variables on demand side for, 34-35; explanatory variables on supply side for, 25-34
Employment: and earnings, trends in, 3-6; of women and ethnic minorities in hospitals, 3
Employment and Earnings (E&E), 3, 6, 126, 127
Estimation, functional form and, 97

Federal Fair Labor Standards Act (1967), 28
Fein, Rashi, 54
Feldman, Roger D., 29, 30, 41-42
Feldstein, Martin, 22, 28, 51, 54, 66, 128; on hospitals as philanthropic wage setters, 6, 7, 14-15, 49, 77
Findings, summary of, 123-127
Fisher, Charles R., 1
Florida, University of, Survey of Hospital Directors of Nursing at, 29

About the Authors

Frank A. Sloan is professor, Department of Economics, and senior research associate, Institute for Public Policy Studies, Vanderbilt University. He received the B.A. from Oberlin College and the Ph.D. in economics from Harvard University. He was a summer intern on the President's Council of Economic Advisors, a Woodrow Wilson National Fellow, and has served as research associate with the Rand Corporation. He has also been a lecturer in the Department of Economics, University of California at Los Angeles, and associate professor, Department of Economics, University of Florida. He serves as a consultant to a number of government and private organizations. Dr. Sloan is coauthor of *Private Physicians and Public Programs* (Lexington Books, 1978.) and *Access to Ambulatory Care and the U.S. Economy* (Lexington Books, 1979).

Bruce Steinwald is research associate and project manager, Institute for Public Policy Studies, Vanderbilt University. He received the B.A. from Johns Hopkins University and the M.B.A. from the University of Chicago Graduate School of Business, where he also completed all requirements except dissertation for the Ph.D. degree. He has been active in health-services research and consulting since the late 1960s, and is currently working with Dr. Sloan on additional research on physicians and hospitals.